Color Atlas and Text of

OSTEOARTHRITIS

Edited by
Michael Doherty
Rheumatology Unit
City Hospital
Nottingham, UK

M Wolfe

Coventry University

Copyright © 1994 Times Mirror International Publishers Limited.
Published in 1994 by Wolfe Publishing, an imprint of Times Mirror International
Publishers Limited.
Copyright Chapter 5 radiographs © 1994 Iain Watt.
Copyright Fig. **7.21** © 1976 American Medical Association.
Printed by Grafos S.A. Arte sobre Papel, Barcelona, Spain.
ISBN 0 7234 1646 X

For full details of all Times Mirror International Publishers Limited titles please write to
Times Mirror International Publishers Limited, Lynton House, 7–12 Tavistock Square,
London WC1H 9LB, England.

A CIP catalogue record for this book is available from the British Library.

Library of Congress Cataloging-in-Publication Data has been applied for.

Contents

Preface

Osteoarthritis (OA) is the commonest condition to affect the joints of man. Over the past 20 years significant advances have been made in our understanding of the biochemistry and anatomic change associated with the condition. The past decade has witnessed increasing interest in the epidemiology, clinical characterisation, imaging, and search for biochemical markers of OA. Now the possibility of modifying the OA process by therapeutic interventions is being discussed. Few books have attempted to encompass the many different aspects of OA, and some that have are now outdated.

This book is intended to give a concise overview of important facets of human OA, with strong emphasis on pictorial presentation. It is not intended as an exhaustive text, but interesting and important data are highlighted. A multidisciplinary approach has been used to ensure balanced perspective, and many of the authors are recognised experts in their field. The book should prove of interest to trainees and specialists in rheumatology and orthopaedics, allied health professionals, and interested general physicians.

Contributors

Peter Bullough
Chief of Pathology
The Hospital for Special Surgery
535 East 70th Street
New York
USA

Timothy Cawston
Head of Research Laboratories
Rheumatology Research Unit
Addenbrooke's Hospital
Hills Road
Cambridge, UK

Cyrus Cooper
MRC Clinical Scientist and Honorary
Consultant Rheumatologist
MRC Environmental Epidemiology Unit
Southampton General Hospital
Southampton, UK

Paul Dieppe
Professor of Rheumatology
Rheumatology Unit
Bristol Royal Infirmary
Bristol, UK

Michael Doherty
Reader in Rheumatology
Rheumatology Unit, City Hospital
Nottingham, UK

Paul Halverson
Associate Professor of Medicine
Department of Internal Medicine
St Joseph's Hospital
5000 W. Chambers
Milwaukee
USA

Charles Hutton
Consultant Rheumatologist
Mount Gould Hospital
Mount Gould Road
Plymouth, UK

Adrian Jones
ARC Clinical Research Fellow
Rheumatology Unit, City Hospital
Nottingham, UK

Joanna Ledingham
Roussel Osteoarthritis Research Fellow
Rheumatology Unit, City Hospital
Nottingham, UK

Ian Leslie
Consultant Orthopaedic Surgeon
Bristol Royal Infirmary
Bristol, UK

Michael Shipley
Consultant Rheumatologist
Bloomsbury Rheumatology Unit
Middlesex Hospital
Authur Stanley House, Tottenham Street
London, UK

Leon Sokoloff
Professor of Pathology
Department of Pathology
Health Sciences Center
State University of New York at Stony Brook
USA

Iain Watt
Consultant Radiologist
Radiology Department
Bristol Royal Infirmary
Bristol, UK

1. Introduction: The Nature of Osteoarthritis

Michael Doherty

Osteoarthritis (OA) is by far the commonest condition to affect the joints of man (Peyron, 1979). It is a major cause of locomotor pain, the single most important rheumatological cause of disability and handicap, and an important health care challenge with major resource implications. Surprisingly, however, OA has only recently become a significant focus of research interest. Its profile is now rapidly changing. Previously considered a 'wear and tear', 'degenerative' disease to be accepted as an inevitable consequence of ageing and trauma, OA is increasingly viewed as a dynamic, essentially reparative process with exciting potential for health intervention.

Terminology: historical perspective

At the turn of the century pathologists and radiologists differentiated two principal forms of chronic arthritis:

- **Atrophic arthritis** with synovial inflammation and erosion or atrophy of cartilage and bone (including several entities such as rheumatoid arthritis).
- **Hypertrophic arthritis**, characterised by focal loss of cartilage, little evidence of inflammation, and by growth (hypertrophy) of adjacent bone and soft tissue (Goldthwaite, 1904).

The latter group became synonymous with **osteoarthritis**. Recognised associations with ageing and joint trauma led to ready acceptance of the alternative term **degenerative joint disease**. In the 1960s and 1970s major research interest increasingly focused on inflammatory arthropathies, with OA often being used in clinical and laboratory studies as a 'non-inflammatory' control, or even as a surrogate for normal joint tissue. Such usage encouraged the term **osteoarthrosis** to emphasise the lack of overt inflammation.

In the past few decades advances in cartilage biochemistry and clinical delineation of polyarticular and crystal-associated subsets proved important catalysts in renewing interest in this condition (Kellgren and Moore, 1952; Lawrence, 1977; McCarty, 1976; McDevitt, et al., 1977; Maroudas, 1979). Although inflammation is not as florid as in 'atrophic' arthropathies, it is undoubtedly a component in many cases (Cooke, 1985), and particularly obvious in some (Ehrlich, 1972), and the term **osteoarthritis (OA)** is generally preferred.

Definition of OA

Concepts of OA are still changing, so it is not a clearly delineated condition. Although there is no universal agreement, a compromise working definition of OA is:

A condition of synovial joints characterised by cartilage loss (chondropathy) and evidence of accompanying periarticular bone response.

Chondropathy may occur without hypertrophic bone response (e.g. polychondritis, rheumatoid), and conversely periarticular new bone may develop without chondropathy (e.g. 'traction' spurs); it is only when both combine in synovial articulations that the term OA is appropriate. Drawbacks of such a definition include:

- Exclusion of joints with early (initial) change.
- Emphasis on cartilage and bone – even though all other joint components (synovium, capsule, entheses, muscle) show changes in OA (**1.1**).
- A structural rather than physiological emphasis – with no consideration of biological consequences (e.g. symptoms, functional impairment).

Nevertheless, given these caveats, such a definition is a practical common starting point for examination of existing epidemiological, clinical and experimental data. The American College of Rheumatology recently devised criteria for classification of symptomatic OA of knee, hip or hand that incorporate both clinical and investigative features in algorithmic form (Altman, 1991). The usefulness of such criteria in population settings and in the context of other spheres of OA interest, however, has yet to be tested.

1.1

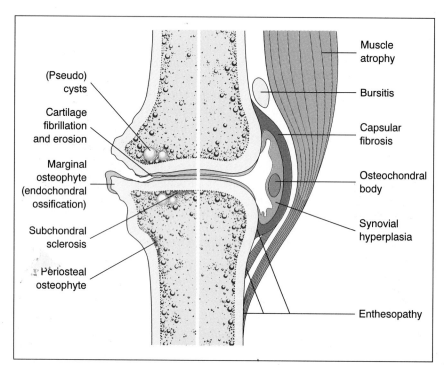

1.1 Joint tissues affected in OA. Commonly emphasised changes (shown on the left) are focal cartilage loss, osteophyte, subchondral sclerosis and 'cysts'. Less emphasised changes (shown on the right) include synovial hypertrophy with contained osteochondral bodies, capsular fibrosis, enthesopathy, bursitis and muscle changes.

The size of the problem

The prevalence of OA is difficult to assess (*see* Chapter 4). Much epidemiological data relate to radiographic changes alone and are problematic in terms of assessment and 'grading', distinction between isolated and chondropathy-associated osteophyte, and relevance to symptoms and function (Peyron, 1979). Nevertheless, although most, if not all, people over the age of 65 years will show structural changes of OA at time of death, the prevalence of symptomatic OA in the UK is estimated in the order of 18:1,000, with a female preponderance and strong age relationship (Wood, 1976; Badley *et al.*, 1978; van Saase *et al.*, 1989). Certainly in terms of use of health care resources, OA is one of the major problems in the developed world (Badley *et al.*, 1978; Kramer *et al.*, 1983). In addition to the burden of severe disability, OA is a common cause of moderate pain and troublesome impairment of mobility in older people (Hadler, 1985). Such problems are increasingly less well tolerated as health education improves and patient expectations increase; inevitable acceptance of the consequences of OA by patients (and doctors) is changing.

The nature of OA

It appears that OA has accompanied man throughout his evolutionary history (Hutton, 1987), and a similar process occurs in other animals that fuse epiphyses in the adult. At the tissue level, chondrocyte, osteocyte, and synoviocyte activities increase in OA, and at certain phases of the process, cell division and biosynthesis may be marked. Radiographic OA is very common in adults, showing increased frequency with age (van Saase *et al.*, 1989); however, in most instances OA occurs without symptoms or disability. Furthermore, symptoms relating to OA are predominantly phasic, and are often associated with a good prognosis (Danielsson, 1964; Danielsson and Hernborg, 1970; Hernborg and Nilsson, 1977; Pattrick *et al.*, 1989).

Such phylogenetic preservation, discordance between symptoms and structural change, biosynthetic activity, and generally good outcome, suggest that OA reflects the inherent repair process of synovial joints (**1.2**). In most cases this metabolically active process keeps pace with a variety of triggering insults and is non-progressive; such 'healing' ability may occasionally be marked (Perry *et al.*, 1972; **1.3**, **1.4**). In some cases, however, it fails to compensate, resulting in 'joint failure' (decompensated OA) with perceived symptoms and disability. This interpretation may in part explain the **marked heterogeneity** of OA, a wide variety of 'insults' triggering a repair reaction (OA) but each resulting in a different pattern of involvement. As with any biological process, multiple constitutional (intrinsic) and environmental (extrinsic) factors may further modify the response, leading to a variable outcome.

As the search for these intrinsic and extrinsic factors continues, it is apparent that:

- Factors relating to **initiation** and **progression** of OA may differ.
- **Different factors** operate at **different joint sites**.
- **Complex interaction** between factors is likely.

The latter has been well illustrated in the knee and the hand. For example, total (particularly lateral) meniscectomy radically alters the biomechanics of the knee and is a recognised predisposing factor for OA of the knee. However, since not all patients develop post-meniscectomy OA such severe mechanical insult alone seems an insufficient cause of OA. The higher frequency and severity of post-meniscectomy OA in individuals predisposed to development of generalised OA strongly supports interaction between local/mechanical and system/constitutional factors in its development (Doherty *et al.*, 1983). A similar interaction is suggested in Blount's disease, in which only a proportion of patients develop knee OA in later life despite possession of severe bilateral varus deformity (Zayer, 1980). The large number of studies investigating occupational or recreational trauma generally concur in showing no great increased risk of OA from repetitive usage or even 'over-usage' of joints; however, local mechanical factors relating to usage may in part determine the site and pattern of development of OA, as elegantly demonstrated in the hands of manual operators in a textile mill (Hadler *et al.*, 1978).

1.2

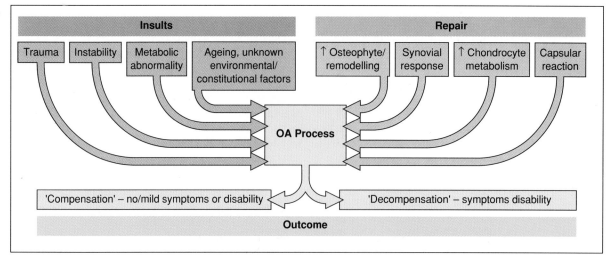

1.2 Diagrammatic representation of OA as a repair process that may be triggered by a variety of insults and show a variable outcome.

1.3

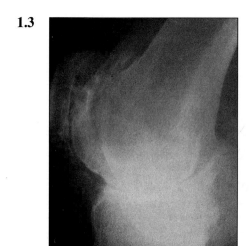

1.4

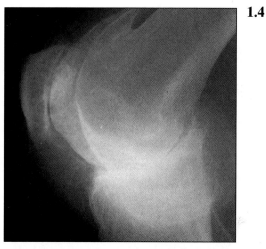

1.3, 1.4 Example of radiographic 'improvement' in a patient with patello-femoral OA. The second film, taken two years after the first, shows osteophyte growth and bone remodelling with clearer definition of bone contours. During this period the patient's symptoms also improved.

OA 'subsets'

Since OA is a process, not a disease, that may be triggered by diverse constitutional and environmental factors, it is not surprising that attempts to define and classify OA as a single disease entity have not been helpful. The trend in recent years has been to separate OA into more homogeneous groupings or 'subsets' in order to define aetiological factors and to determine natural history and prognosis.

OA was initially classified as **primary** (no cause identified) or **secondary** (an obvious cause identified, such as trauma or dysplasia; **1.5**, **1.6**). However, such artificial separation often proved unsatisfactory for the following reasons:

- Frequent lack of an identifiable cause, resulting in a large still heterogeneous primary group.
- Frequent overlap between subsets (Doherty *et al.*, 1983).

In addition to identifiable predisposing factors, other more objective features have therefore often been used as a further basis of subset differentiation. For example:

- The joint **site** involved (hip, knee, hand).
- The **number** of joints involved – one, few, many (Kellgren and Moore, 1952).
- The **pattern of involvement** – between and within joints (Kellgren and Moore, 1952; Solomon, 1983).
- The presence of **associated crystal deposition** (McCarty, 1976; Doherty and Dieppe 1988; **1.7**).
- The presence of marked clinical **inflammation** (Ehrlich, 1972).
- The radiographic bone response (**atrophic, hypertrophic**) (Solomon, 1983; **1.8**, **1.9**).

In practice, some 'subsets' have emerged which differ in a number of such characteristics. It is important to note, however, that sharp distinction between subsets does not exist. Many of the above characteristics represent different aspects of the OA process (the balance between damage and repair), and may dominate the clinical picture at just one phase in the evolution of the condition. One subset may thus evolve into another, and different subsets may exist at different sites within the same individual. Possibly the most important distinction is simply by site and number of joints involved; predisposing factors are increasingly being associated with specific joint sites, or with polyarticular as opposed to pauci-articular involvement.

1.5

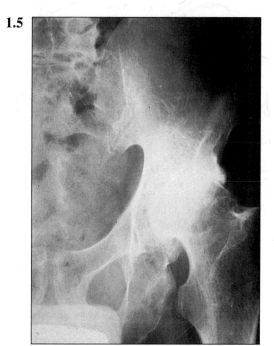

1.6

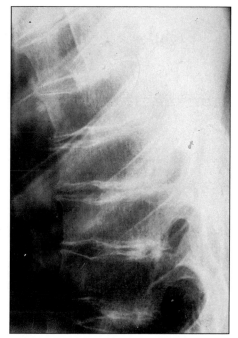

1.5, 1.6 Spondylo-epiphyseal dysplasia causing 'secondary', premature OA in a 34-year-old man.

1.7

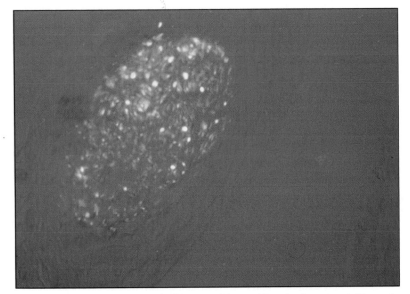

1.7 Calcium pyrophosphate crystal deposition evident in the synovial/capsule biopsy of a patient with OA of knee.

1.8

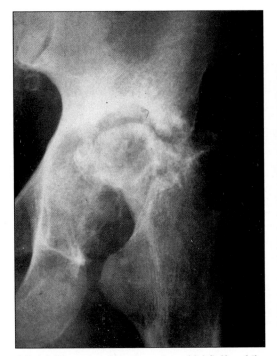

1.9

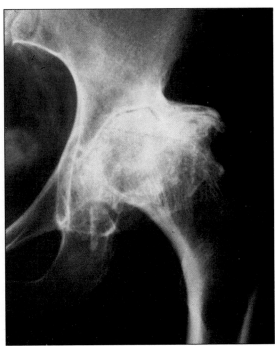

1.8, 1.9 Comparison between an 'atrophic' (left) and 'hypertrophic' (right) pattern of OA of hip.

Problems related to the study of OA

OA has proved a very difficult condition to study, for both clinicians and basic scientists alike. Several of the major problems are listed in **Table 1.1.** The lack of agreed criteria and definitions, and poor correlation between clinical and pathological features have already been emphasised. OA is age-related and it develops and changes very slowly; this makes it difficult to follow the condition over any length of time, and to identify early changes. There are still very few markers or measurements of the process, and outcome measures are poor. Problems of the appropriateness of animal models of OA mean that few data, if any, can be extrapolated to the human situation. Finally, the heterogeneity of the disorder is particularly problematic, and means that knowledge concerning pathogenesis, risk factors, or treatment success of OA cannot necessarily be extrapolated from one joint site to another.

Despite these difficulties, considerable progress is now being made with respect to the understanding of biochemical and histological changes in OA, the identification of risk factors, and approaches to treatment. Indeed, the past decade has witnessed increasing interest in the possibility of pharmacological intervention to modify aspects of this repair process and thus improve outcome – a consideration that would not have been entertained just a few years ago. Why OA is at last being viewed as an interesting condition will become apparent in forthcoming chapters, which overview important aspects of the OA process and provide current interpretation of recent highlighted advances.

Table 1.1 Some difficulties relating to the study of OA.

Lack of clear definition of the condition

Lack of agreed diagnostic criteria

Poor correlation between X-rays and clinical features

Slow, age-related changes

No suitable process measures

Poor outcome measures

Difficulties with animal models of 'OA'

Heterogeneity of clinical expression and outcome

References and further reading

Altman, R.D. (1991) Criteria for classification of clinical osteoarthritis. *J. Rheumatol.*, **18** (Suppl. 27), 10–12.

Badley, E.M., Thompson, R.P., Wood, P.H.N. (1978) The prevalence and severity of major disabling conditions. *Int. J. Epidemiol.*, **7**(2), 145–151.

Cooke, T.D.V. (1985) Pathogenic mechanisms in polyarticular osteoarthritis. *Clin. Rheum. Dis.*, **11**(2), 203–238.

Danielsson, L.G. (1964) Incidence and prognosis of coxarthrosis. *Acta Orthop. Scand.*, (Suppl. 66), 1–114.

Danielsson, L.G. and Hernborg, J. (1970) Morbidity and mortality of osteoarthritis of the knee (gonarthrosis) in Malmo, Sweden. *Clin. Orthop. Rel. Res.*, **69**, 224–226.

Doherty, M. and Dieppe, P.A. (1988) Clinical aspects of calcium pyrophosphate dihydrate crystal deposition. *Rheum. Dis. Clin. N. Am.*, **14**, pp. 395–414.

Doherty, M., Watt, I., and Dieppe, P. (1983) Influence of primary generalised osteoarthritis on development of secondary osteoarthritis. *Lancet*, **ii**, 8–11.

Ehrlich, G.E. (1972) Inflammatory osteoarthritis: I. The clinical syndrome. *J. Chron. Dis.*, **25**, 317–328.

Goldthwaite, J.E. (1904) The differential diagnosis and treatment of so-called rheumatoid diseases. *Bost. Med. Surg. J.*, **151**, 529–534.

Hadler, N. (1985) Osteoarthritis as a public health problem. *Clin. Rheum. Dis.*, **11**(2), 175–185.

Hadler, N.M., Gillings, D.B., Imbus, H.R., Levitin, P.M., Makuc, D., Utsinger, P.D., Yount, W.J., Slusser, D., and Moskovitz, N. (1978) Hand structure and function in an industrial setting. Influence of three patterns of stereotyped repetetive usage. *Arthritis Rheum.*, **21**, 210–220.

Hernborg, J.S., Nilsson, B.E. (1977) The natural course of untreated osteoarthritis of the knee. *Clin. Orthop. Rel. Res.*, **123**, 130–137.

Hutton, C. (1987) Generalised osteoarthritis: an evolutionary problem. *Lancet*, 1463–1465.

Kellgren, J.H., Moore, R. (1952) Generalised osteoarthritis and Heberden's nodes. *Br. Med. J.*, **1**, 181–187.

Kramer, J.S., Yelin, E.H., Epstein, W.V. (1983) Social and economic impacts of four musculoskeletal conditions; a study using national community-based data. *Arthritis Rheum.*, **26**, 901–907.

Lawrence, J.S. (1977) *Rheumatism in Populations*. Heinemann Medical Books, London.

Maroudas, A. (1979) Physiochemical properties of articular cartilage. In *Adult Articular Cartilage*, Freeman, M.A.R. (Ed.), Pitman, London, pp. 215–290.

McCarty, D.J. (1976) Calcium pyrophosphate dihydrate crystal deposition disease – 1975. *Arthritis Rheum.*, **19** (suppl.), 275–286.

McDevitt, C., Gilbertson, E., Muir, H. (1977) An experimental model of osteoarthritis: early morphological and biochemical changes. *J. Bone Joint Surg.*, **59B**, 24–35.

Pattrick, M., Aldridge, S., Hamilton, E., Manhire, A., Doherty, M. (1989) A controlled study of hand function in nodal and erosive osteoarthritis. *Ann. Rheum. Dis.*, **48**, 978–982.

Perry, G.H., Smith, M.J.G., Whiteside, C.G. (1972) Spontaneous recovery of the joint space in degenerative hip disease. *Ann. Rheum. Dis.*, **31**, 440–448.

Peyron, J.G. (1979) Epidemiologic and aetiologic approach to osteoarthritis. *Sem. Arthritis Rheum.*, **8**, 288–306.

Solomon, L. (1983) Osteoarthritis, local and generalised: a uniform disease? *J. Rheumatol.*, **10** (suppl. 9), 13–15.

van Saase, J.L.C.M., van Romunde, L.K.J., Cats, A., Vandenbrouke, J.P., Valkenburg, H.A. (1989) Epidemiology of osteoarthritis: Zoetermeer survey. Comparison of radiological osteoarthritis in a Dutch population with that in 10 other populations. *Ann. Rheum. Dis.*, **48**, 271–280.

Wood, P.H.N. (1976) Osteoarthritis in the community. *Clin. Rheum. Dis.*, **2**(3), 495–507.

Zayer, M. (1980) Osteoarthritis following Blount's disease. *Int. Orthop.*, **4**, 63–66.Figure 1.1

2. The Epidemiology of Osteoarthritis

Cyrus Cooper; Paul Dieppe

Osteoarthritis (OA) remains an enigmatic condition to the epidemiologist. It is probably the most common joint disorder to afflict western populations, yet there is no consensus as to its definition. The aetiology, clinical features and natural history remain obscure, and the generation of effective preventive strategies to limit its impact seems a distant goal. In this chapter three aspects of the epidemiology of OA are reviewed:

- Approaches to the definition and classification of the disorder.
- Descriptive epidemiology.
- Individual risk factors and their relevance to aetiological hypotheses.

The definition and classification of OA

Definition

The subdivision of arthritic conditions, with the notable exception of acute gout, into discrete disease entities is a relatively recent phenomenon. In the first decade of this century, pathologists and radiologists differentiated between two broad types of arthropathy: atrophic and hypertrophic. The former were characterised by synovial inflammation with erosion of cartilage and bone, the latter by primary cartilage damage with hypertrophy of subchondral bone. The atrophic form came to be subdivided further, into septic arthritis, rheumatoid arthritis and ankylosing spondylitis, as advances were made in microbiology and rheumatology. Hypertrophic arthritis, however, was never further subdivided, and over the years the term became synonymous with the condition now called OA. This term therefore encompasses a large and heterogeneous spectrum of idiopathic joint disorders.

Thus no simple definition of OA exists. Any working definition of the disorder will entail consideration of pathological, radiological and clinical components (**2.1**).

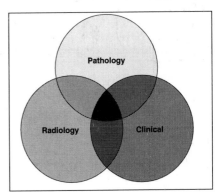

2.1

2.1 The definition of OA. The term requires consideration of three broad areas: pathological changes, radiographic appearances and clinical consequences.

Pathology

The key feature of OA at the tissue level is focal destruction of articular cartilage (**2.2**). Cartilage is composed of a matrix, the three major constituents of which are collagen, proteoglycans and water, which provide it with its important functional properties of smooth articular motion and shock absorption. The chondrocyte, the cell type responsible for synthesis and degradation of cartilage, lies within this matrix. Under normal circumstances, a dynamic equilibrium is maintained between cartilage synthesis and breakdown. The earliest pathological finding in OA is disruption of the collagen meshwork, resulting in fissuring of the articular cartilage. There is progressive focal erosion and ulceration at some sites, associated with cell necrosis. Attempts at cartilage repair take the form of chondrocyte proliferation at adjacent sites and the formation of disordered reparative cartilage.

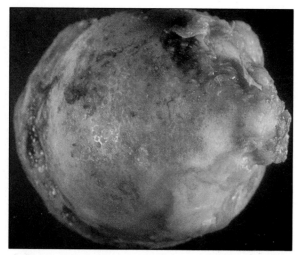

These cartilage changes are followed by changes in subchondral bone. Denudation of cartilage increases the local stress borne by the underlying bone, which sustains focal microfractures. Increased intra-articular pressure may result in cyst formation in areas of weakened bone. These injuries are followed by reparative changes within the bone itself: subchondral new bone formation, which results in bony sclerosis, and osteophyte formation, in an attempt to buttress the joint margins.

2.2 Excised femoral head from a patient with OA of the hip. Note extensive loss of articular cartilage with eburnation of subchondral bone. (Reproduced with kind permission of the publishers, Gower Medical.)

Radiology

The radiographic features conventionally used to define and assess the severity of OA include joint space narrowing, osteophyte formation, subchondral sclerosis, cyst formation and abnormality of bony contour. These features purport to measure various pathological changes which occur in cartilage and subchondral bone as a result of OA (**Table 2.1**). Recent evidence, however, suggests problems with both the validity and reproducibility of several of these radiographic features (**2.3–2.5**). Their distribution in the general population, the relationships between them and their clinical significance remain for the most part unknown.

Despite these limitations, most epidemiological studies of OA have adopted a five-point radiographic scale for grading the severity of the condition which was devised more than 30 years ago (**Table 2.2, 2.6**). This scale relates to an atlas of standard radiographs which are used for assessments at various joint sites. Particular inadequacies of the system are the emphasis placed upon the osteophyte, and the assumption implicit in the scale that radiographic progression of OA follows a single, predictable course. Both of these tenets have been recently challenged. Nevertheless, much of the data drawn upon in the later part of this chapter relate to OA defined radiographically according to this system.

Table 2.1 The association between pathological changes in OA and accompanying radiographic features.

Pathology	Radiology
Cartilage loss	Joint space narrowing
Bone formation	Osteophyte Subchondral sclerosis
Vascular engorgement and high turnover	Cyst
Disrupted trabecular architecture	Deformity

Table 2.2 Radiographic criteria for the assessment of OA (Kellgren and Lawrence).

Grade 0	None	No features of OA
Grade 1	Doubtful	Minute osteophyte, doubtful significance
Grade 2	Minimal	Definite osteophyte, unimpaired joint space
Grade 3	Moderate	Moderate diminution of joint space
Grade 4	Severe	Joint space greatly impaired with sclerosis of subchondral bone

3

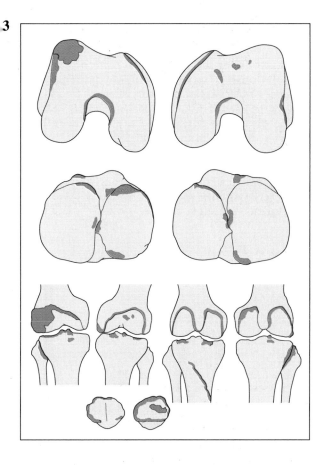

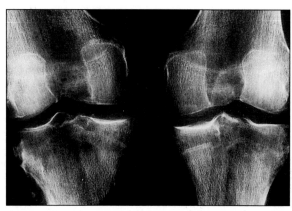

2.4

2.3, 2.4 Problems in the radiographic definition of OA – validity. This palaeopathological specimen from a man dying around 1450 shows extensive osteophytosis around the femoral condyles, with eburnation (indicated on **2.3** in red and blue respectively). The accompanying radiograph (**2.4**) reveals changes which are much less marked. (Reproduced with kind permission of Dr Juliet Rogers.)

2.5

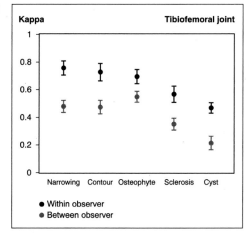

2.5 Problems in the radiographic definition of OA – reproducibility. Diagrammatic representation of between and within observer reproducibility for five widely used radiographic features of OA. A kappa statistic of 1.0 indicates perfect concordance of paired readings, while one of 0 indicates concordance no greater than that expected by chance alone. Certain features (e.g. joint space narrowing) are considerably more reproducible than others (e.g. sclerosis and cyst).

2.6

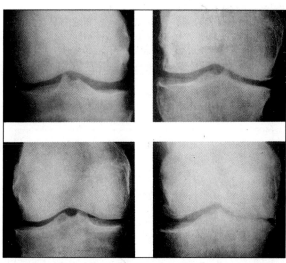

2.6 Radiographic criteria for the assessment of OA devised by Kellgren and Lawrence for the Empire Rheumatism Council. The radiographs show Grades 1 to 4 (reproduced from the *Atlas of Standard Radiographs* with kind permission of the publishers, Blackwell Scientific).

Clinical

Two broad clinical areas are relevant to any definition of OA. First, the symptoms associated with the condition, and second, the degree and characteristics of the disability which constitute its longer term sequelae.

Joint pain is the dominant symptom of OA. In the general population the prevalence of joint pain rises markedly with age. A recent survey of knee pain in a population sample of elderly British people showed a prevalence rising from around 20% at age 55 years to over 30% in women aged 85 years (**2.7**). The association, however, between joint pain and radiographic features of OA is not constant. In studies performed during the 1950s in the north of England, the relationship between pain and radiographic evidence of OA was considerably stronger for the hip than for the knee or distal interphalangeal joint (**2.8**).

The disability attributable to OA is even less precisely defined. In the survey described above, a relationship was found between reported knee pain and disability at all ages and in both sexes (**2.9**). However, both disability and OA rise in frequency with age, and the presence of other sources of morbidity make such observations difficult to interpret.

2.7

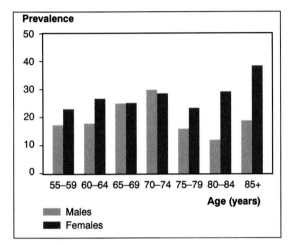

2.7 The prevalence of knee pain in the elderly population. These data were obtained from a postal questionnaire survey of 2,000 people aged 50 years and over in Bristol (reproduced with kind permission of Dr T. McAlindon).

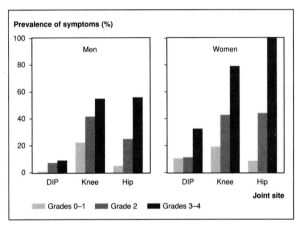

2.8 Discordance between symptoms and radiographic changes in OA. The data were derived from population surveys in northern England (Lawrence, 1977). They show the variable relationship between joint pain and radiographic grade of OA at the distal interphalangeal joint (DIP), knee and hip.

2.9

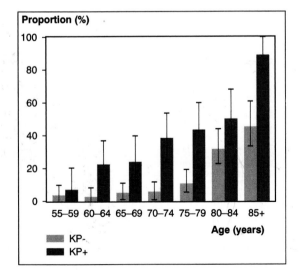

2.9 Knee pain and disability among elderly men and women. The graph shows that disability (measured using the modified Standford Health Assessment Questionnaire) is strongly associated with knee pain (KP) in an elderly population sample (*see* **2.7**; reproduced with kind permission of Dr T. McAlindon).

Classification

Several systems for the classification of OA have been proposed.

Aetiological

The recognition that pathological and radiological features of OA could follow almost any established joint disorder led to the proposition that OA might be classified as primary or secondary. Secondary OA could follow a host of conditions including inflammatory arthritis, metabolic disorders, crystal deposition and developmental abnormalities (**Table 2.3**).

Table 2.3 The classification of osteoarthritis according to aetiology.

1. Primary (no known cause)

2. Secondary

–   to pre-existing joint disease:
  • Rheumatoid arthritis
  • Septic arthritis
  • Gout
  • Paget's disease
  • Hyperparathyroidism
  • Avascular necrosis

–   to metabolic or systemic predisposition:
  • Ochronosis
  • Haemachromatosis
  • Chondrocalcinosis
  • Acromegaly
  • Hypermobility

–   to local mechanical factors:
  • Trauma
  • Meniscectomy
  • Developmental disorders (Perthes' disease)

Pathological

Subchondral bone responses vary from the formation of huge masses of new bone at joint margins (hypertrophic) to the absence of any response with bone destruction (atrophic). There is some evidence that hip OA can be separated into different categories, with different associations and prognosis, on this basis (**2.10, 2.11**). The recognition of inflammatory (**2.12**) and erosive (**2.13**) subsets of OA is another example of such classification.

2.10

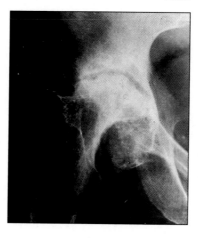 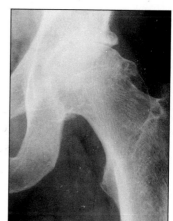

2.11

2.10, 2.11 Atrophic (**2.10**), and hypertrophic (**2.11**) OA of the hip. The radiograph on the right shows cartilage loss with marked subchondral bony reaction and exuberant osteophytosis. The radiograph on the left shows little bony reaction with predominant bone attrition. There is some evidence that the natural history of these two variants is different, with hypertrophic disease being relatively stable over long periods of time, but atrophic change being rapidly progressive. (Reproduced with kind permission of Professor L. Solomon.)

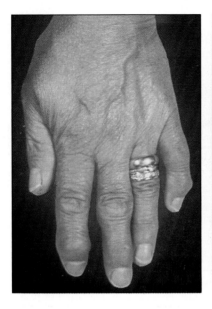

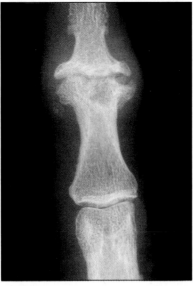

2.12 Inflammatory OA. This post-menopausal woman had warm, red, tender swellings at the distal inter-phalangeal and proximal inter-phalangeal joints, radiographic features of OA and a moderate rise in inflammatory indices. (Reproduced with kind permission of the publishers, Gower Medical.)

2.13 Erosive OA. Note cartilage loss with subarticular erosions.

Articular

Just as there is great heterogeneity in the effects and manifestations of OA at one joint, there is great variation in the pattern of affected joint distribution in different individuals. The main sites involved are shown in **2.14**. There is a particular predilection for the distal interphalangeal joints of the hand, the thumb base, knee, hip and intervertebral facet joint. Involvement of more than one joint is common, and many population surveys have reported that subjects with OA in one joint have a frequency of OA in other joints which cannot be explained by chance or age alone. In 1952, Kellgren and Moore described the condition of generalised osteo-arthrosis, in which Heberden's nodes were associated with polyarticular OA. They found that first-degree relatives of probands with generalised osteoarthrosis had twice the expected prevalence of multiple joint involvement, and confirmed the hereditary nature of this diathesis in a twin study.

In hospital practice in the UK, three major subsets of OA may be discerned on the basis of pattern of joint involvement:

• Knee/hand OA.
• Isolated hip OA.
• Polyarticular OA.

These patterns are not clear-cut or mutually exclusive. The picture of OA which emerges is that of a balance between two processes: a systemic predisposition to involvement of many joints within a certain distribution, and local mechanical factors which predispose to joint failure at individual sites.

In summary, the term OA has various facets. At the pathological and radiological levels, components of the osteoarthritic process reflect damage and repair to differing degrees. The impact of these processes on joint symptoms and disability is not clearly understood. Although these difficulties in definition have undoubtedly constrained epidemiological research into OA, population-based radiographic surveys have provided some data on the occurrence and risk factors for the condition.

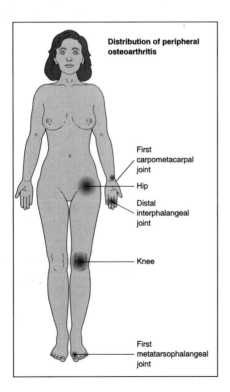

2.14

Distribution of peripheral osteoarthritis

First carpometacarpal joint
Hip
Distal interphalangeal joint
Knee
First metatarsophalangeal joint

2.14 Peripheral joint distribution of OA.

The descriptive epidemiology of OA

Pathological features

Autopsy studies have assessed the prevalence of cartilage abnormalities and OA in people who have died of other diseases. Prevalence estimates from such studies tend to be higher than those from radiographic surveys, perhaps because the whole joint surface is available for examination. Almost universal evidence of cartilage damage has been reported by one investigation in people aged over 65 years. In another, cartilage erosion, subchondral bony reaction and osteophyte were found in the knees of 60% of men and 70% of women who died in the seventh and eighth decades of life. The prevalence of advanced disease was 17% in men and 38% in women, rising to 58% over the age of 85 years.

Radiographic surveys

Several radiographic surveys of OA have been performed. The largest and most comprehensive of these included 6,585 subjects studied between 1975 and 1978 in the suburban Dutch district of Zoetermeer (van Saase *et al.*, 1989). As with most such studies, radiographic assessment used the Empire Rheumatism Council Atlas of Standard Radiographs.

Data from this survey are used here to depict the major epidemiological characteristics of OA at three joint sites: the distal interphalangeal (DIP) joint, knee and hip. These sites have been chosen as they illustrate differences in their pattern of occurrence with age and sex (**2.15–2.17**).

2.15

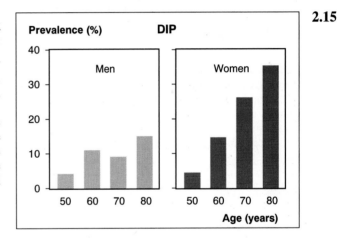

2.16

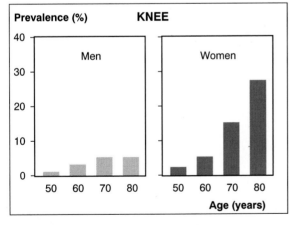

2.17

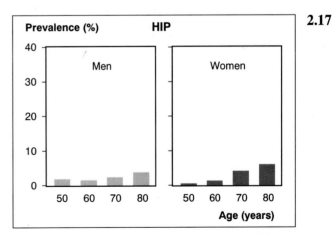

2.15–2.17 The prevalence of OA in the distal interphalangeal joint, knee and hip, in a large population-based Dutch survey (after van Saase *et al.*, 1989).

Age

Age is a major determinant of the prevalence of OA at all three of these joint sites. Over 60% of men and women aged 70 years and over had evidence of mild (Grade 2) or severe (Grades 3 and 4) OA in the DIP joint. This was the most frequent joint site to be involved, followed by the first metatarsophalangeal joint of the foot. OA of the knee and hip were found to be less frequent. All three sites showed a tendency to increased prevalence of OA with advancing age, and this trend occurred in men and women.

Sex

When all joint sites are amalgamated, there appears to be little or no overall sex difference in the prevalence of mild OA. A female preponderance becomes more apparent, however, for severe grades of OA, in older age groups, and for OA of the hand and knee.

Ethnic group

The prevalence of OA of the hands and feet has been assessed in several different ethnic groups (**2.18**). The condition has been reported in all the populations examined, and rates are remarkably consistent given the difficulties of representative sampling and reproducible radiographic assessment. A different picture emerges for OA of the hip (**2.19**) which appears to have a substantially lower prevalence among Negroid and Oriental populations than among Caucasians. These differences have been attributed to variation in the reported frequency of mild acetabular dysplasia in these populations.

2.18

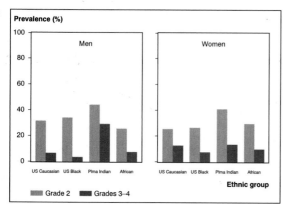

2.19

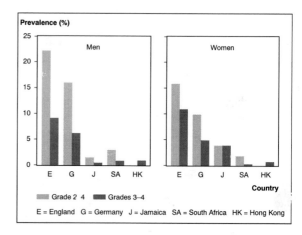

2.18 Ethnic variation in the prevalence of OA in the hands and feet (after Lawrence and Sebo, 1980).

2.19 Geographic variation in the prevalence of hip OA (after Felson, 1988).

Individual risk factors for OA

The individual risk factors for OA may be conveniently viewed as acting through two major pathogenic mechanisms:

- Factors influencing or marking a generalised predisposition to the condition.
- Factors resulting in abnormal biomechanical loading at specific joint sites (**2.20**).

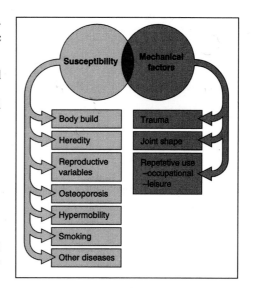

2.20 Individual risk factors for OA. The two broad pathogenic mechanisms are a generalised predisposition to the condition, and local mechanical factors.

Generalised susceptibility

Obesity

Adiposity is closely associated with osteoarthritis at the DIP joint and knee, but less so with osteoarthritis of the hip. Population-based studies suggest that the increase in risk of knee OA between highest and lowest fifths of the distribution of body mass index (BMI) lies between four- and seven-fold (**2.21**). Until recently, it was not clear whether obesity preceded (and perhaps caused) OA, or whether obesity resulted from the sedentary lifestyle of patients with OA. Two pieces of evidence now suggest that the former assertion is correct. First, analysis of the Framingham epidemiological study in the USA has revealed that obesity predicted subsequent knee OA up to 30 years later. Second, analysis of HANES data has shown that obesity is consistent in its association with both symptomatic and asymptomatic OA.

The reason for the association between obesity and OA remains speculative. Although mechanical loading appears an attractive mechanism at first sight, it does not explain the differential effects of adiposity at the hip (small effect), hand and knee (large effect). Some studies point toward a stronger association in women than in men. Thus metabolic, rather than mechanical, factors may be more important in the pathogenesis of the disorder.

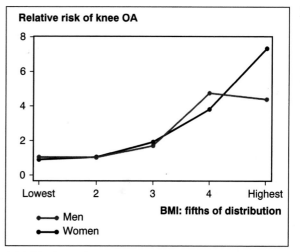

2.21 Obesity and the risk of knee OA. Data are derived from the Health and Nutrition Examination Survey in the United States (HANES, after Felson, 1988).

Heredity

As evidenced by generalised OA (see p. 20).

Reproductive variables

The marked female predominance of polyarticular OA has led many commentators to suggest that this clinical subgroup is hormonally mediated. The disorder appears to increase in prevalence after the menopause in women, and OA has been associated with previous hysterectomy. Oestrogen receptors have recently been identified on the osteoblast surface, and *in vitro* studies have suggested that female sex hormones modify chondrocytes in culture conditions. Attempts to retard the development of OA using postmenopausal hormone replacement therapy, however, have generally been unsuccessful.

Osteoporosis

OA at particular sites also appears to have a negative association with osteoporosis. The strongest evidence for this lies at the hip joint, where studies consistently observe that elderly patients with hip OA are at lower risk of sustaining femoral neck fractures. In patients with polyarticular disease, studies of bone density have produced inconsistent results. Here, much of the difference in bone density between patients with OA and controls may be explained by the association of the disorder with obesity. The osteoarthritis–osteoporosis relationship, if real, supports the view that abnormal mechanical behaviour of subchondral bone underlies accelerated cartilage damage. Certainly in rare inherited bone diseases such as osteopetrosis, where the skeleton is diffusely sclerotic, there is a high incidence of premature polyarticular OA (**2.22**).

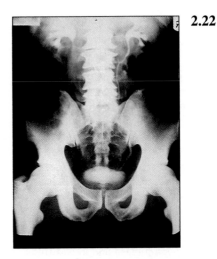

2.22

2.22 OA (marble bone/Albers–Schönberg disease). An inherited disorder in which generalised bony sclerosis occurs in the skeleton. OA is a frequent sequel, and may result from abnormal load-bearing properties of subchondral bone. (Reproduced with kind permission of Dr Iain Watt.)

Hypermobility

The range of motion of any joint has a normal distribution in the population. Generalised ligamentous laxity, the prerequisite of joint hypermobility (**2.23**), is therefore seen in a substantial proportion of healthy people. Hypermobility diminishes rapidly throughout childhood and then more slowly during later life. Women are more mobile than men, and Asians more mobile than Caucasians. Generalised joint laxity is a feature of several rare inherited disorders of collagen, such as Ehlers–Danlos syndrome. Hypermobility in the absence of identifiable collagen gene abnormalities may result in a wide variety of overuse lesions, as well as osteoarthritis. The strength of the association with osteoarthritis, as well as its precise mechanism, remain subjects for further study.

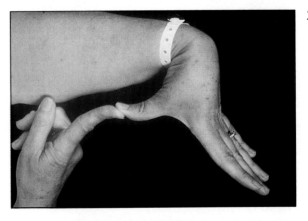

2.23

2.23 The hypermobility syndrome. The ability to reach the forearm with the thumb on wrist flexion suggests joint laxity. The condition may be associated with OA.

Cigarette smoking

Analysis of one large population-based data set suggests that cigarette smoking has a protective influence on the development of OA. This effect remained after adjustment for potential confounding variables, but needs confirmation.

Other diseases

Associations have been documented between OA and diabetes mellitus, hypertension and hyperuricaemia, which are independent of obesity. The association with diabetes may have particular aetiological significance through the increased prevalence of diffuse idiopathic skeletal hyperostosis (DISH), or Forestier's disease, in this condition.

Mechanical factors

Trauma

Major injury is a common cause of knee OA. Two specific types of injury are associated: cruciate ligament damage and meniscal tears (**2.24**, **2.25**). Follow-up studies of patients with cruciate rupture (particularly when bilateral), have reported cartilage loss, even in young patients. For meniscectomy, most studies have reported an increased frequency of subsequent OA. The risk rises with advancing age, presence of a generalised predisposition to OA (as evidenced by Heberden's nodes) and time since meniscectomy. Major injury, particularly fracture, may alter mechanical function and predispose to OA at other sites. Most notable among these are fractures of the femoral shaft (hip OA), tibia (ankle OA), humerus (shoulder OA) and scaphoid (wrist OA).

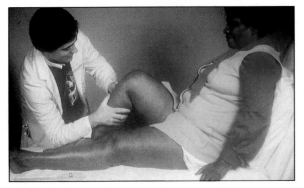

2.24 Rupture of the cruciate ligaments. Detected by the anterior and posterior draw signs, the condition predisposes to knee OA. (Reproduced with kind permission of Dr T. McAlindon.)

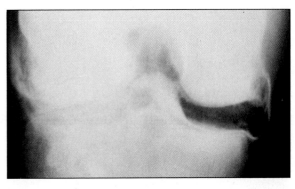

2.25 Meniscectomy. This arthrogram of a patient who previously had a meniscectomy shows marked loss of articular cartilage. (Reproduced with kind permission of Dr I. Watt.)

Joint shape

The sites at which joint shape has been most closely linked with later development of OA are the hip and knee. It is well established that childhood hip disorders such as Perthes' disease, slipped capital epiphysis and congenital dislocation of the hip lead to premature hip OA (**2.26**). It is also likely that milder degrees of acetabular dysplasia account for some cases of hip OA among younger subjects (**2.27, 2.28**). However, the impact of this mild developmental abnormality in causing later hip OA remains questionable.

It has also been proposed that dysplasia of the femoral condyles alters the biomechanical stability of the knee joint and predisposes to OA (**2.29**).

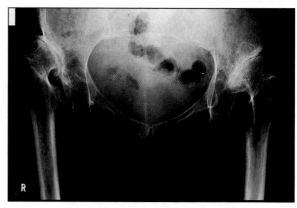

2.26 OA of the hip following congenital dislocation.

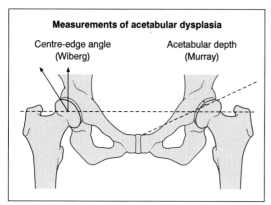

2.27 The measurement of acetabular dysplasia. Wiberg's centre-edge angle and Murray's acetabular depth are the most frequently used measures of this disorder which may account for some cases of hip OA in later life.

2.28

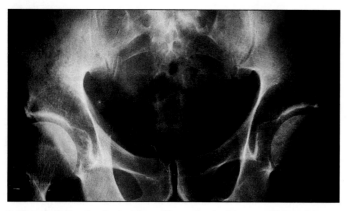

2.28 Acetabular dysplasia. The radiograph of a 34-year-old Spanish woman, with reduced acetabular depth and centre edge angle.

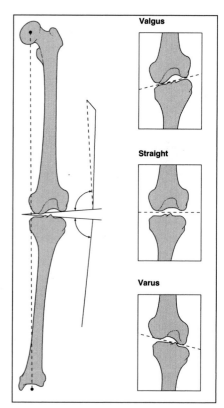

2.29 Knee dysplasia and OA. The diagram on the left illustrates the normal angulation of the left femur on the tibia and the load line passing medial to the knee joint. The diagrams on the right show that variable dysplasia of the medial and lateral femoral condyles will result in valgus or varus deformity. These deformities may predispose to OA of the knee.

Occupation

Occupational activity exemplifies stereotyped repetitive use of particular joint groups. The association of hand OA with handedness, and the relatively infrequent involvement of paretic limbs by the condition point to a role for repetitive activity in the aetiology of OA. Several occupational groups have been shown to be at increased risk of developing OA (**Table 2.4**). Elegant studies have suggested that the localisation of OA to particular joint groups in the hands of cotton workers are related to the specific activities they perform in the workplace. Recent data from the Health and Nutrition Examination Survey in the USA also suggest an association between repetitive knee use in the workplace and OA at this site.

Table 2.4 Occupational groups at increased risk of OA.

Occupation	Joint group affected
Miners	Hip, knee, shoulder
Dockers	Hip, knee
Welders	Knee
Foundry workers	Elbow
Cotton workers	Hands
Farmers	Hip
Forestry workers	Hip

Leisure physical activity

Sporting activity combines the risks of major joint damage with those of repetitive use. In sports associated with significant trauma, such as American football, there appears to be a high incidence of ensuing lower limb OA. The association between moderate physical activity and the risk of OA remains uncertain.

Summary

OA is a clinically heterogeneous, multifactorial disorder, which has certain constant pathological and radiological features. The incidence and risk factors for the condition are best treated separately at different joint sites, although strong evidence has accumulated for certain patterns of joint involvement (such as the association between hand and knee disease). The pathogenesis depends upon the interplay between a generalised susceptibility to OA, and local mechanical imbalance at particular joints. A greater understanding of its epidemiology will hasten the delineation of effective population-based preventive strategies.

References and further reading

Felson, D.T. (1988) Epidemiology of hip and knee osteoarthritis. *Epidemiol. Rev.*, **10**: 1–28.

Grahame, R. (1990) The hypermobility syndrome. *Ann. Rheum. Dis.,* **49**: 199–200.

Kirwan, J.R., Silman, A.J. (1987) Epidemiological, sociological and environmental aspects of rheumatoid arthritis and osteoarthritis. *Baillières Clin. Rheumatol.*, **1**: 467–489.

Lawrence, J.S. (1977) *Rheumatism in populations.* Heinemann Medical Books, London.

Lawrence, J.S., Sebo, M. (1980) The geography of osteoarthritis. *In:* Nuki, G.(ed.). *The aetiopathogenesis of osteoarthritis.* Pitman Medical, London, 155–183.

Peyron, J.G. (1984) The epidemiology of osteoarthritis. *In:* Moskowitz, R.W. *et al.* (eds.). *Osteoarthritis: diagnosis and management.* W.B. Saunders, Philadelphia, 9–27.

The epidemiology of chronic rheumatism. Vol. 2. Atlas of standard radiographs. Blackwell Scientific Publications, Oxford, 1963.

van Saase, J.L.C.M., van Romunde, L.K.J., Cats, A., Vandenbroucke, J.P., Valkenburg, H.A. (1989) Epidemiology of osteoarthritis: Zoetermeer survey. Comparison of radiological osteoarthritis in a Dutch population with that in 10 other populations. *Ann. Rheum. Dis., 48,* 271–280.

Acknowledgements

We thank the Arthritis and Rheumatism Council for financial support.

3. Pathology and Biochemistry of Osteoarthritis

Peter Bullough; Timothy Cawston

Acute disease is the result of acute malfunction and is the consequence of injury either mechanical trauma, infection, or metabolic abnormalities. Acute disease may become chronic as a result of continuing injury or ineffective or imperfect repair. In connective tissues, acute injury may lead to profound and immediate malfunction (eg. fracture of bone) and the processes of repair will restore normal function only if normal anatomy is restored.

Since there is no agreed definition of osteoarthritis (OA), the following is offered: "OA is a functional disorder of joints, characterized by altered joint anatomy, especially the loss of articular cartilage. Unlike many other forms of arthritis, it is not obviously inflammatory." It may be unhelpful to regard OA as a distinct entity. Rather, it may result from a number of different pathophysiological pathways.

Some of the questions which have been asked about OA are:

- Is OA a single disorder or a family of disorders?
- What are the roles of acute and chronic trauma in pathogenesis?
- Is OA an inevitable consequence of aging?
- How do the anatomical, physiological, biochemical, and mechanical alterations in cartilage matrix interrelate in the pathogenesis of OA?
- What roles do extra cartilaginous structures play in the disease?
- Under what circumstances does significant microscopic evidence of inflammation develop?
- Does articular cartilage repair in OA?

This chapter will attempt to address these questions by considering the physiology and anatomy of the normal joint, and relating them to the pathophysiology and morbid anatomy of the diseased joint.

The normal joint

Function

Normal joint function is characterized by:

- The freedom of the opposed articular surfaces to move painlessly over each other within the required range of motion.
- A proper distribution of load across joint tissues which could otherwise be damaged by overloading or fail to be maintained because of habitual underloading (disuse).
- The maintenance of stability during use.

These interdependent aspects of joint function themselves depend on three features of joint anatomy:

- The shapes of the joint surfaces need to be very precisely matched. Firstly, to permit the necessary range of motion. Secondly, to provide stability and thirdly, to provide as wide and as equitable loading as possible during use.
- The connective tissue matrices which provide the mechanical properties; these are both synthesized and broken down by their intrinsic cells, i.e. osteoblasts, osteocytes, osteoclasts and chondrocytes (Schenk *et al.*, 1986). To maintain the physicochemical and mechanical properties of tissues, these cell functions must be subject to highly sensitive feedback systems as yet poorly understood.
- The ligaments, muscles and tendons supporting the joint and of the nervous system which controls them. (A standard animal model used in research to study developing OA is created by sectioning the anterior cruciate ligament of a knee. (Moskowitz, 1992 ; McDevitt *et al.*, 1977)

Shape

The most obvious feature of any joint is its shape with one joint surface essentially convex, while the other is concave. The convex side of the joint generally has a larger articular surface than the concave side. In some joints, for example, in the hip and the ankle, the articular surfaces appear at first sight to make a very exact fit (i.e., they appear congruent) and for a long time it was considered that a precise fit or congruency, was a normal feature of a joint (Hammond and Charnley, 1967). However, in other joints (e.g. knee and finger joints), the surfaces appear quite incongruent. In many joints, the gross incongruencies of the opposed surfaces are partially corrected by interposed pliable intra-articular fibro-cartilaginous menisci (e.g. knee) (Bullough, 1970).

Both cartilage and bone undergo elastic deformation under load. As load increases, the surfaces of the joint come into increasing contact, and so spread the load over the articular cartilage and the underlying bone equitably. The incongruity and the deformation of the joint space under load provide for the circulation and mixing of the synovial fluid essential to the metabolism of the chondrocytes (**3.1, 3.2**).

3.1

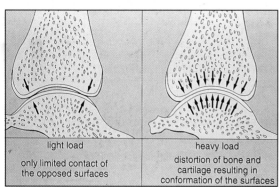

light load

only limited contact of the opposed surfaces

heavy load

distortion of bone and cartilage resulting in conformation of the surfaces

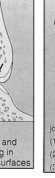

joint shape provides for
(1) movement
(2) load distribution
(3) stability

3.2

3.1, 3.2 Elastic deformation under load.

Materials

The expanded cancellous bone end is covered by articular cartilage which is tethered to the jagged surface of the underlying bone by a thin layer of interlocking calcified cartilage (**3.3, 3.4**). The extracellular matrix of cartilage is composed of three substances:

- Collagen, a fibrous protein that provides strength and form to cartilage.
- Proteoglycans, a glycoprotein 'stuffing material' found between collagen fibrils that confers stiffness and elasticity to cartilage.
- Water (up to 80% of the weight of the cartilage), which contributes to cartilage turgor.

This functional matrix is synthesized and maintained by a small number of cells which although representing less than 1–2% of the total volume of the cartilage are responsible for maintaining tissue integrity.

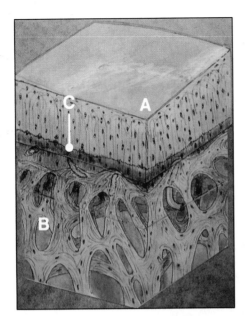

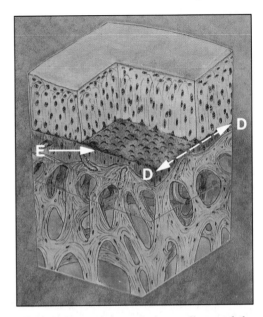

3.3, 3.4 Two drawings which demonstrate the relationship between the articular cartilage and the underlying bone. The cartilage (A) is locked into the underlying bone (B) by a thin layer of calcified cartilage (C). The mineralization front of the calcified cartilage or 'tidemark' (D) is marked by a basophilic line, and chondrocytes embedded within it regulate its advance into the non-calcified articular cartilage. The invasion of blood vessels from the marrow space into the calcified cartilage (E) slowly replaces it with bone through the process of endochondral ossification.

Chondrocytes

The chondrocytes embedded in the cartilage matrix, are responsible for synthesis and maintenance of the tissue. They vary in size, shape and number of cells per unit volume of tissue both from the surface to the deeper layers and in different anatomic locations. Generally, cells at the cartilage surface are flatter, smaller and orientated parallel with the cartilage surface. These cells are surrounded by a network of fine collagen fibrils and this region is less rich in proteoglycans. They also have a greater density than the cells deeper in the matrix (Stockwell, 1979). In the middle zones, chondrocytes are more spherical, and arranged in columns. This vertical arrangement of cells probably reflects some interaction with collagen fibres. The highly organized arrangement of collagen fibres in cartilage suggests the possibility of movement of chondrocytes within the matrix substance as the collagen is being laid down. In adult human cartilage, chondrocytes do not obviously proliferate except in response to disease and injury.

Chondrocytes are surrounded by a specialized matrix distinctly different from the bulk of extracellular matrix. Immediately surrounding the chondrocytes is a matrix rich in proteoglycans and some hyaluronic acid but relatively little collagen. Around this is a basket like structure composed of cross-linked fibrillar collagen encapsulating the cell or sometimes groups of cells and this provides a protective framework. Collagen Type VI is found in this region.

Mitochondria are sparse in chondrocytes, probably relating to their comparatively low rates of oxygen consumption. Cells in the deeper uncalcified zone have the most prominent endoplasmic reticulum as Golgi apparatus indicating active protein synthesis as well as sulphation of proteoglycan carbohydrate side chains. The cell membrane shows numerous short as well as some longer, branched cytoplasmic processes, but they make no connection with the processes of other chondrocytes. In the extracellular matrix adjacent to the cells of adult articular cartilage, as in the hypertrophic zone of the growth place, small membrane-bound vesicles are visible. These may play an important role in calcification of cartilage matrix (Anderson, 1980).

An interesting ultrastructural feature of chondrocytes is a non-motile monocilium which may have a mechanotransductory function in regulation of matrix synthesis (Wilsman, 1978).

Collagen

Fourteen different types of collagen are now known (Van der Rest 1991). All contain the classical triple helix (**3.5**). These molecules vary in size. Some contain interrupted helix structures aligned in a staggered array to form collagen fibrils. The classic banded appearance of collagen is caused by regions of overlap or gaps in the packing of the molecules.

Hyaline cartilage has a unique type of collagen, Type II, which is structurally characterized by three triple helical alpha-1 (II) chains. The Type II fibrillar network is essential for maintaining the tissues volume and shape giving articular cartilage its tensile strength. Individual collagen molecules are cross-linked by strong pyridinoline-type cross links (Eyre 1992) (**3.6**).

Electron-microscopic studies show that in the surface layer collagen fibres are closely packed, of fine diameter, and mostly oriented parallel to the joint surface (Bullough and Goodfellow, 1968).

The collagen content of cartilage progressively diminishes from the superficial to the deep layer (Muir *et al.*, 1970). In deeper layers, collagen fibres are more widely separated, thicker in diameter, and are vertically aligned in such a fashion as to form a web of arch-shaped structures (**3.7**). The fibres are continuous with those in the calcified layer of cartilage, but not with underlying subchondral bone. The arrangement of arches allows collagen to constrain the proteoglycan gel entrapped in the matrix. The web of arches functions as a unit, and damage to one section can be expected to affect the architectural integrity of the whole unit.

In addition to Type II collagen, cartilage also contains a number of collagens which although present at low concentration nevertheless perform vital functions. Type IX collagen belongs to a group of fibril associated collagens and has an interrupted triple helix, a large globular domain and a covalently linked glycosaminoglycan chain which may act as a linkage between the Type II collagen network and proteoglycans (**3.8**). This collagen appears to bind the surface of Type II collagen fibres and limits their size. The proportion of Type IX collagen therefore may play a major role in modulating the mechanical properties of cartilage. Also present is Type XI collagen. This fibre forming collagen (**3.9**) is found within the interior of the Type II collagen fibrils and is thought to organize surrounding collagen Type II molecules during fibrillogenesis. Type X collagen is a non-fibrillar collagen found in calcifying cartilage restricted to matrix around hypertrophic chondrocytes of the growth plate and in the deep calcified zone (Mayne and Irwin, 1986) (**3.10**).

3.5

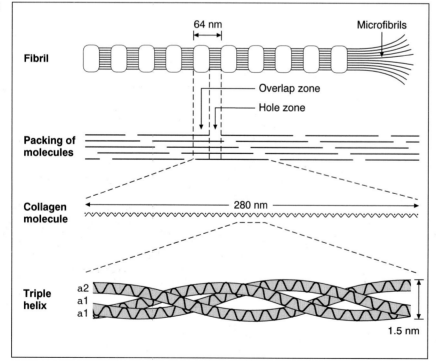

3.5 Structure of collagen. Three amino acid coils are wound around each other to produce the very stable triple helical structure of collagen. These molecules then associate in a staggered array, leaving gaps and overlap regions, which gives rise to the classic banded appearance of collagen fibres.

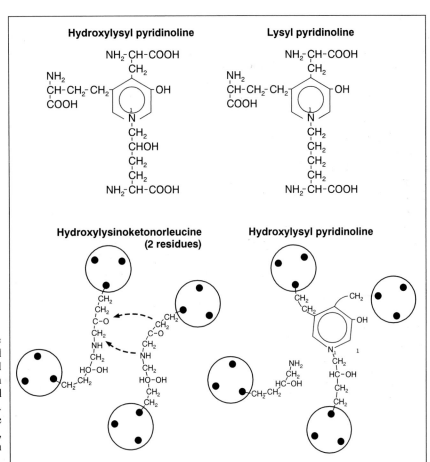

3.6

3.6 Collagen crosslinks. The collagen fibres are stabilized and their tensile strength is increased by crosslinks that form between different regions of the staggered array of triple helical molecules. Crosslinks form via OH-Lysine residues along the collagen chain, and the structures of two such crosslinks are shown.

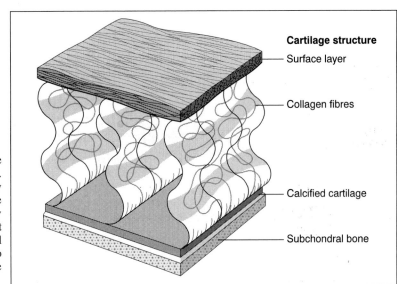

3.7

3.7 The collagen fibres in cartilage are arranged in a characteristic pattern. Fibres rise vertically in a leaf-like array from the calcification front, but change to a horizontal orientation as they approach the surface. This arrangement contains the PG molecules as they pull water into the tissue and swell, and also protect the chondrocytes that are embedded in the matrix.

3.8

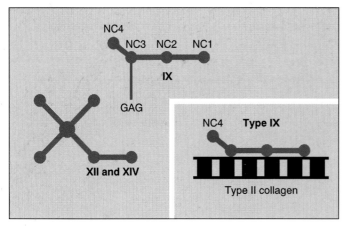

3.8 Fibril associated collagens. Type IX collagen found in cartilage contains four non-collagen domains and has an attached GAG chain. It is thought to bind to the surface of the Type II collagen fibre and limit its growth.

3.9

TYPE	MOLECULES	REPRESENTATIVE TISSUES
I	$[\alpha 1(I)]_2 \alpha 2(I)$	skin, bone, tendon, dentin etc.
	$[\alpha 1(I)]_3$	dentin, skin (minor form)
II	$[\alpha 1(II)]_3$	hyaline cartilage, vitreous body
III	$[\alpha 1(III)]_3$	skin, vessels
V	$[\alpha 1(V)]_3$	hamster lung cell cultures
	$[\alpha 1(V)]_2 \alpha 2(V)$	foetal membranes, skin, bone
	$\alpha 1(V)\alpha 2(V)\alpha 3(V)$	placenta, synovial membranes
XI	$\alpha 1(XI)\alpha 2(XI)\alpha 3(XI)$	hyaline cartilage

3.9 Fibre forming collagens. Type II and Type XI collagens both form fibres and are found in articular cartilage. Type XI collagen is thought to be responsible for initiating the formation of the Type II fibres.

3.10 Non-fibre forming collagens. Type X collagen is one of a group of collagen molecules that do not form fibres that are shown in this figure. It consists of three Type X α chains and is found in the growth plate. It is thought to be present where calcification of cartilage occurs and is often found around hypertrophic chondrocytes.

TYPE	MOLECULES	REPRESENTATIVE TISSUES
IV	$[\alpha1(IV)]_2\alpha2(IV)$	basement membranes
VI	$\alpha1(VI)\alpha2(VI)\alpha3(VI)$	vessels, skin, invertebral disc
VII	$[\alpha1(VII)]_3$	dermoepidermal junction
VIII	(?)	Descemet's membrane, endothelial cells
IX	$\alpha1(IX)\alpha2(IX)\alpha3(IX)$	hyaline cartilage, vitreous humour
X	$[\alpha1(X)]_3$	growth plate (hypertrophic cartilage)
XII	$[\alpha1(XII)]_3$	embryonic skin and tendon, periodontal ligament
XIII	(?)	endothelial cells
XIV	$[\alpha1(XIV)]_3$	foetal skin and tendon

Proteoglycans

Proteoglycans (PGs) are a diverse group of heterogenous molecules consisting of protein chains and attached carbohydrates. The large, hydrated proteoglycan molecules are found filling in the spaces between and are loosely attached to, the collagen fibrils (Rosenberg and Buckwalter, 1986).

In contrast to the fibrous structure of collagen, proteoglycan is a sticky gel-like molecule. The major proteoglycan in cartilage is aggrecan, containing a protein core of Mr 215000 to which carbohydrate side chains (keratan and chondroitin sulphate) are attached. The core protein contains three globular domains and two extended interglobular domains (**3.11**). At the N-terminal end, the first globular domain interacts with hyaluronic acid and this interaction is stabilized by link protein. As many as 200 aggrecan molecules (monomers) bind to one hyaluronic acid chain (Mr 1-2 $\times 10^6$) to form an aggregate (Mr 5×10^7 to 5×10^8) hence the name aggrecan (Hascall, 1988). PGs are highly charged molecules and attract water and swell considerably. However, the expansion of the PGs is restricted to approximately 20% of the maximum possible by the collagen network and this creates a swelling pressure. When cartilage is loaded, some water is extruded and PGs are compressed. Removal of the load permits the imbibing of water into the tissue together with essential nutrients until the swelling pressure of the PGs is balanced by the resistance of the collagen network. Aggrecan shows an age related decrease in size and an enrichment in keratan sulphate relative to chondroitin sulphate or protein content. These changes reflect changes in PG synthesis and also extracellular cleavage by proteinases (Thonar and Kuettner, 1987).

In addition to aggrecan, cartilage contains other PGs containing dermatan sulphate. Two PGs called biglycan and decorin differ in size (Mr approximately 98000 and 68000 respectively), core protein structure and properties. These PGs are present in low concentrations and show increasing concentration with age especially in superficial layers (Bianco et al., 1990). They also interact with other proteins in the extracellular matrix (**3.12**). Decorin is located on the surface of collagen fibers and inhibits collagen fibril formation. They appear to inhibit processes involved in tissue repair and may have a role in preventing joint adhesions. A further PG like molecule fibromodulin, with keratan sulphate side chains, is located on the surface of collagen fibrils (**3.13**).

Articular cartilage also contains other extracellular matrix proteins (Heinegard et al., 1992). Chondrocalcin is a protein probably involved in the calcification process. Anchorin is a protein on the surface of chondrocytes involved in binding of these cells to extracellular matrix components possibly transmitting altered stress on Type II fibres to chondrocytes. Fibronectin, thrombomodulin, cartilage oligomeric high Mr matrix protein are all found in cartilage but their precise functions are not yet known. The possible arrangement of all these components within the cartilage matrix is shown schematically in **3.12**.

The topographic distribution of these PGs exhibits a great deal of local variation within the cartilage matrix which may reflect local mechanical requirements (Bjelle, 1975).

3.11

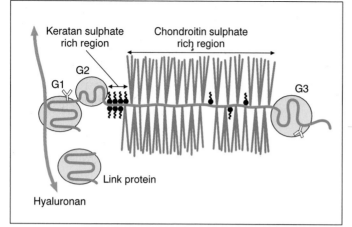

3.11 Structure of aggrecan. The PG aggrecan is made up of a polypeptide chain with three globular domains G1-G3 interspersed with extended regions to which are attached sulphated glycosaminoglycan side chains, keratan and chondroitin sulphate. G1 associates with hyaluronic acid in association with link protein. Up to 200 aggrecan molecules can associate with hyaluronic acid to form a large molecular aggregate that is highly charged, and pulls water into the tissue.

3.12

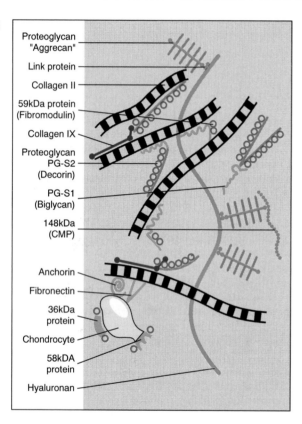

3.12 Association of the different cartilage components. The figure illustrates the possible interactions of the different molecules found in cartilage.

Tissue heterogeneity

Heterogeneity of cartilage tissue including biochemical, morphological and biomechanical variations, can be observed within different regions of a normal weight-bearing joint. Maroudas *et al.*, (1973) observed topographical variations in PG content in the cartilage of the femoral head. Kempson *et al.* (1970) further observed that variation in stiffness seen in different areas of the femoral head was related to PG content and to the amount of water held by the tissue.

An example of normal geographic variation can be observed in the tibial plateau, of man as well as other animals, where there are distinct morphological differences between articular cartilage which is covered and that which is not covered by the meniscus. These differences consist of a rough surface and soft matrix in the uncovered area compared to the smooth, firm areas covered by the meniscus. Bennett *et al.* (Bennett and Waine, 1942) reported that all individuals over 16 years showed focal roughening of the uncovered cartilage on the tibial plateau. We have also examined adult human as well as dog knee joints at autopsy and found that articular cartilage not covered by meniscus always showed matrix softening and superficial fibrillation. The morphologic and biochemical findings in these two distinct articular areas as studies in the adult dog are summarized in Bullough *et al.*, 1985 (see **3.13**).

Naturally occurring variations in matrix structure and mechanical properties may be related to joint loading (Tammi *et al.*, 1987). In the normally functioning knee, load is transmitted through the meniscus and onto the tibial cartilage underlying the meniscus, whereas the exposed cartilage, that which is not covered by the meniscus, remains relatively unloaded (Bullough and Walker, 1977). Similar areas of possible disuse atrophy, have been described around the rim of the radial head, (Goodfellow and Bullough, 1967) in the roof of the acetabulum and on the perifoveal and inferomedial aspects of the femoral head (Bullough *et al.*, 1973).

3.13 Summary of morphology and biochemistry. **Left:** In the covered area, the surface is smooth, there is an amorphous electron-dense layer, and cells are flattened. With respect to lipid, there is an increased intracellular accumulation in all three layers, there is an increased extracellular accumulation at the surface, and there are increased numbers of extracellular matrix vesicles in the deep zone. Collagen appears in randomly oriented fibers with thicker mean diameters, there is regular binding of proteoglycan, and the concentration per wet weight is increased. Proteoglycan shows an increased concentration per wet weight. The tidemark is irregular. **Right:** In the uncovered area, the surface is irregular, there is a detached electron-dense layer, and cells are rounded. The concentration of water per unit volume is increased. Collagen appears in wavy aggregated bundles with thinner mean diameters (small range), and binding of proteoglycan is ill defined. An increased amount of proteoglycan can be extracted. The tidemark is smooth. In both the covered and the uncovered areas, the cell size is the same histologically and there is the same amount of DNA per dry weight of cartilage tissue.

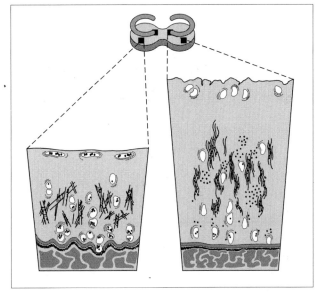

3.13

Linkage

Functional joint anatomy must include consideration of the ligaments and tendons joining articulating surfaces and surrounding the joint, as well as the neuromuscular control of joint motion. Sensory feedback monitors our movements through the modalities of touch, temperature, pain, and position sense. Proper joint function depends on intact ligaments and neuromuscular coordination. As recognized by Charcot in the nineteenth century, a breakdown of neuromuscular coordination can lead to profound arthritis.

Little is known about the changes that occur in tendons and ligaments that surround the joint during the development of OA but it is interesting that early changes in cartilage as seen by MRI are often accompanied by changes in the tendon and ligaments surrounding the joint. It is important to note that the current overemphasis on cartilage as the only tissue affected by OA needs to be tempered with a wider approach that considers all the affected structures within the joint.

Physiology

Normal function requires maintenance of joint shape and cartilage tissue.

Joint shape

This is mostly determined by bone not the cartilage. While the general shapes of joint surfaces are genetically determined, maintenance of the functional shape of a particular joint depends on environmental forces acting upon it. The shape of the bone, including the articular ends, is maintained by feedback mechanisms dependent on mechanical stress to maintain a joint shape capable of distributing load optimally [Wolff's law].

Both growth and modelling occur by enchondral ossification. This process is exemplified in the epiphyseal growth plate where calcified cartilage is invaded by blood vessels from subchondral bone and is replaced by bone tissue synthesized by osteoblasts in close proximity to blood vessels.

Studies of adult joints have shown that replacement of the calcified layer of articular cartilage by bone also occurs through this process. Replacement of calcified cartilage by new bone might be expected to result in cartilage thinning and eventual disappearance. However, histological study of cartilage of various ages shows that this does not happen, both calcified and non-calcified cartilage remaining much the same thickness throughout life. However, the calcification front continues to advance into the non-calcified cartilage at a slow rate in equilibrium with the rate of absorption of calcified cartilage from the subchondral bone. Therefore, articular cartilage is not a static tissue, as it was long thought to be. The matrix and cartilage cells are formed throughout life as the joint is continuously remodelled.

The number of blood vessels entering the calcified articular cartilage and the rate of enchondral ossification change with age; they generally decline up to the age of 60 years and then increase in old age to levels comparable to those of youth (Lane *et al.*, 1977). This change in modelling activity of the joint could reflect an increased need for compensatory remodelling resulting from a loss of joint stability in older individuals due to neuromuscular degeneration. Anatomical studies have supported the view that subtle changes in the shape of a joint occur with age and the examination of radiographs of the joints of young and old adults will show that the joint of an older person is deeper and more angular in its outline that of a young healthy adult (**3.14**).

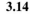 **3.14**

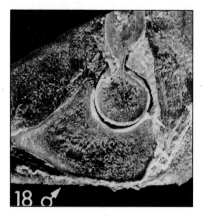

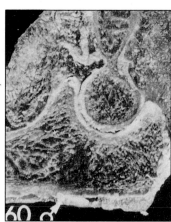

3.14 A sagittal section through the humero-ulnar joint in an 18-year-old, as compared with a 60-year-old. Not only is the joint somewhat deeper in the 60-year-old, but there is a loss of the incongruity that characterized the young joint.

In adult articular cartilage the calcification front (tidemark) is marked histologically by a well-defined line (**3.15**) and contains lipid, ATPase and alkaline phosphatase. A marked change in proteoglycan content of the matrix at the tidemark is demonstrated both by histochemical staining and biochemical analysis (Boskey *et al.*, 1980). These findings indicate specific cellular activity in the region of the tidemark, implying a regulation process.

When the tidemark is examined using scanning electron microscopy (Bullough and Jagannath, 1983) chondrocytes are embedded in the surface of the calcification front and around each is a small mound of calcified tissue (**3.16**). The cellular distribution at the calcification front suggests that the process of calcification is dependent on chondrocytes.

Studies of endochondral ossification in epiphyseal growth cartilage have suggested that calcification is an active process initiated in extracellular membrane-bound vesicles, 0.1–0.2 micrometers in diameter, in proximity to the chondrocytes. In a similar fashion, the physiological calcification of articular cartilage at the tidemark is an active process and histological examination shows that the cells are viable and active and also associated with the presence of extracellular matrix vesicles (Boskey, 1979). Calcification at this site is not, except in some pathological states, a passive process following death of the cell (i.e. not dystrophic calcification).

The feedback mechanisms which control formation and advancement of the calcification front are poorly understood although it appears they are related to loading. Cells close to the calcification front produce substances that promote mineralization. These include extracellular matrix vesicles that provide sites for hydroxyapatite deposition (Ali *et al.*, 1971), enzymes that increase local calcium and phosphate concentration (Matsuzawa and Anderson, 1971; Felix and Fleisch, 1976; Fortuna *et al.*, 1979), phosphoproteins (Leaver *et al.*, 1975), glycoproteins (Termine *et al.*, 1981), proteolipids (Boyan-Salyers, 1980), and calcium phospholipid complexes (Boskey, 1978). All of these may be involved in the initial mineral deposition. In addition, there are other factors that regulate the size and orientation of mineral crystals and inhibit or limit the extend of calcification. These inhibitory substances include proteoglycans (Blumenthal *et al.*, 1979), nucleotide triphosphate and pyrophosphate (Blumenthal *et al.*, 1977).

The concept of continuous growth and remodelling of the articular ends of bone by sustained endochondral ossification is not new. This concept advanced by Ogston (1876) remained dormant until Johnson and others readvanced the idea of continuous remodelling based upon the study of the temporomandibular joint in the human adult (Johnson, 1964).

3.15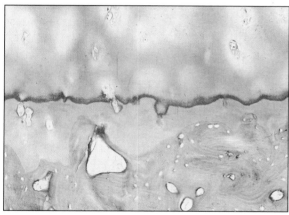

3.15 A photomicrograph to show the relationship between the articular cartilage and the underlying subchondral bone. The calcification front or tidemark, which demarcates the thin layer of calcified cartilage adjacent to the bone from the overlying hyaline cartilage, is marked by a well-defined basophilic line (× 4).

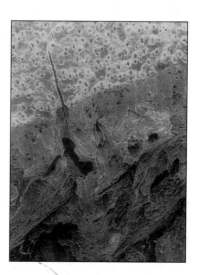 **3.16**

3.16 A scanning electron photomicrograph of the calcified cartilage and underlying subchondral bone. The majority of the cartilage, which is not calcified, has been digested away with hydrazine to expose the surface of the tidemark. The small holes, which are seen in the surface of the tidemark, were occupied by chondrocytes. Around each one of the chondrocyte lacunae, there is a piling-up of calcium salts.

Materials

The extracellular matrix of the cartilage as well as of the other connective tissues is synthesized by their intrinsic cells under the control of both environmental and genetic factors. Both *in vivo* and well as *in vitro* studies have demonstrated that environmental changes result in altered cartilage matrix (Caterson and Lowther, 1978; Lippielo *et al.*, 1985). Immobilization or unloading of a joint results in decreased synthesis of PGs whilst exercise appears to increase synthesis (Palmoski *et al.*, 1979). *In vivo* studies using both cell and organ culture systems have studied the effects of intermittent loading, and of continuous loading both in compression and tension (Veldhuijzen *et al.*, 1979; Jones *et al.*, 1982; Palmoski and Brandt, 1984; DeWitt *et al.*, 1984; Van Kampen *et al.*, 1985). In general, it seems that with low ranges of mechanical stress, that is below the physiologic range, there is enhanced catabolic activity whilst in the physiological range there is anabolic activity. With higher stresses than those in the physiological range the chondrocytes are unable to adapt. In other words, there is a physiological window of stress outside of which, either too low or too high, the chondrocytes are unable to maintain an adequate functions matrix (**3.17**).

Although a number of substances especially cAMP, (Kosher and Savage, 1980), and cytokines including prostaglandin E2 (Houston *et al.*, 1982) have been implicated in the transduction of mechanical stimuli to metabolic events, their role still remains unclear.

3.17

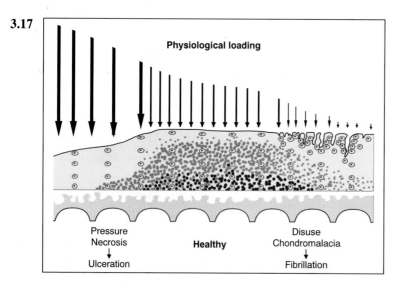

3.17 Diagram illustrating the effect of load on cartilage morphology. Excess load produces cell death and matrix degeneration. Too little load results in alterations in the proteoglycans and the accumulation of water, resulting in chondromalacia. Functional cartilage depends upon normal loading patterns. (This illustration is adapted from The Pathophysiology of Bone and Joint Disease by Teitelbaum and Bullough, a teaching monograph published by *American Journal of Pathology* 1979, Vol. 196, No. 1, p. 335(53)).

The osteoarthritic joint

Clinical arthritis is the consequence of a breakdown in the joint's normal function which in turn is associated with altered anatomy. There is loss of freedom for the articulating surfaces to move over one another easily and a loss of joint stability. The loss of freedom of motion is associated with: loss of articular cartilage, a change in joint shape, and alterations in the ligamentous support and neuromuscular control. Pain may have its origin in the bone, as a result of maldistribution of load, or from the synovium, as a result of reactive synovitis, or may result from muscle spasm.

Malfunction of a joint may result from acute or chronic injuries that produce either anatomical alterations in the shape of the articulating surfaces; or loss of integrity of the support structures around the joint; or alterations in the mechanical properties of the tissue matrices making up the joint (bone, cartilage, synovium, ligaments).

Morbid anatomy

Shape

A change in shape, resulting from cartilage and bone loss, is characteristic of most forms of arthritis. However, in OA, though bone and cartilage loss play an important part in the process, it is the addition of new bone and cartilage in the form of osteophytes, particularly at the joint periphery, although sometimes beneath the articular surface, which forms one of the characteristic feature of the disease.

In each joint the location of osteophytes is characteristic. In the distal interphalangeal joints, osteophytes are prominent on the dorsal and palmar aspects of both articulating surfaces. In the metatarsal-phalangeal joint of the big toe, the osteophyte is on the medial joint margin (hallux valgus). In the hip joint, although osteophytes are generally present around the whole of the joint margin, there is characteristically a large flat osteophyte on the medial articular surface which extends to the fovea (Macys *et al.*, 1980) (**3.18**). Despite the loss of bone and cartilage in some parts of the joint, the net effect of new bone formation is an overall increase in joint size. The osteoarthritic joint is, in general, larger than its normal counterpart.

The osteophytes form by endochondral ossification in one of two ways. Firstly, by vascular penetration into existing cartilage. In these areas, cartilage overlying the bony outgrowth is generally hypercellular, and the process resembles histologically the epiphyseal growth plate in the growing animal (**3.19**). Frequently, in the base of the osteophyte there are remnants of the original tidemark and zone of calcified cartilage and in some cases these remnants are themselves undergoing ossification not only from the region of the original subchondral bone but also from the osteophyte itself (**3.20**). Osteophytes may also form from foci of cartilaginous metaplasia at the joint margins. These foci of metaplasia occur at the capsular and ligamentous insertions (Moskowitz and Goldberg, 1987) and in some instances are at some distance from the joint margin (as on the medial aspect of the femoral neck).

In areas of residual cartilage on the articular surface of a diseased joint there is often marked reduplication and irregularity of the tidemark with histologic evidence of increased endochondral ossification expanding the subchondral bone periphery without actually forming an osteophyte. The microscopic evidence for increased endochondral ossification is, an increased irregularity of the bone cartilage junction, increased vascular penetration of the calcified cartilage and the laying down of woven (immature) bone at the bone cartilage interface (**3.21**).

A slight degree of cartilage reduplication is present in all joints in particular anatomic locations especially at the periphery of joints and beneath prominent ridges on the joint surface, for example, the lateral ridges that define the patello-femoral joint on the surface of the femur. However, in the OA joint, tidemark reduplication is much more widespread and is particularly evident beneath areas of surface erosion and fibrillation. In these areas, the tidemark is generally more irregular, thickened, very distinct and often 3–4 or even more parallel tidemarks can be discerned (**3.22**).

3.18

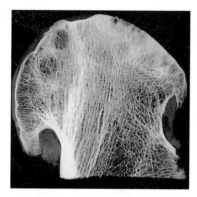

3.18 A radiograph of a 3mm coronal slice through an arthritic femoral head demonstrates the typical medial osteophyte beneath which can still be seen the original outline of the femoral head. Note how the loss of bone from the superior portion of the head is apparently balanced by the addition of new bone medially, thus tending to preserve the sphericity of the head.

3.19

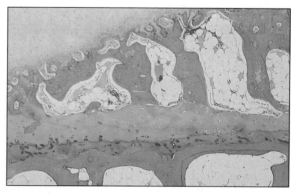

3.19 Photomicrograph to demonstrate the formation of an osteophyte. Note that the articular cartilage overlying osteophyte is more cellular than that of the original cartilage lying between the osteophyte and the subchondral bone. Active endochondral ossification is seen at the junction of the cellular cartilage and osteophytic bone (× 4).

3.20

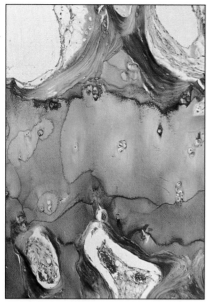

3.21

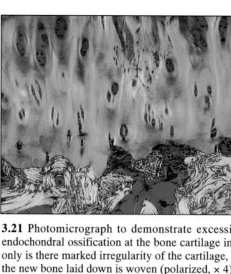

3.21 Photomicrograph to demonstrate excessively active endochondral ossification at the bone cartilage interface. Not only is there marked irregularity of the cartilage, but much of the new bone laid down is woven (polarized, × 4).

3.20 A photomicrograph to demonstrate residual cartilage between subchondral bone below and osteophytic bone above. A mineralization front is seen on both sides of the trapped residual cartilage. Endochondral ossification is occurring on both sides, which will eventually result in the disappearance of the residual cartilage.

3.22

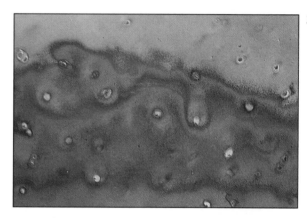

3.22 A photomicrograph to demonstrate tidemark replication.

Tissue

Whatever the cause of injury, certain basic cellular and tissue responses occur. Macroscopically and microscopically there will be evidence of both degeneration and regeneration repair. In connective tissues, there are alterations both in the cells and extracellular matrix. Those in the extracellular matrix may result from direct physical injury, or from enzymatic breakdown, or from alteration in the cellular synthesis of the matrix. In non-vascularized tissue, such as cartilage, an inflammatory response and subsequent scarring cannot occur, but this does not preclude tissue regeneration.

Cartilage injury and repair
Macroscopic changes

Naked-eye evidence of injury to cartilage is seen only in the extracellular cartilage matrix, mainly the collagenous component. One of the earliest findings is disruption of the surface which becomes rough and/or eroded. There are three patterns of macroscopic alteration involving the cartilage surface and to a variable degree the underlying cartilage tissue; fibrillation, erosion and cracking.

Fibrillation describes a surface that appears similar to that of cut velvet. It occurs on both thick cartilage (patella) and thin cartilage (interphalangeal joint). The "pile" of the fibrillated area may be short or shaggy. The junction between the fibrillated area and adjacent normal cartilage is well defined and generally distinct.

Although areas of fibrillation occur in normal cartilage designated by Byers et al. (1970) as "non-progressive lesions" (**3.23**) in osteoarthritic joints, there are areas of fibrillation which appear to be secondary to prior erosion of the cartilage surface. The microscopic characterization of these two distinct types of fibrillation, is incomplete, but perhaps the latter is distinguished by deeper clefts and a greater tendency to form cartilage clones.

Cartilage erosion is characteristic of progressive degenerative changes in the joint. The base of the erosion appears initially to be either contoured or smooth. In knee joints dissected at autopsy from elderly subjects, erosions are found characteristically under the posterior horn of the lateral meniscus and may be related to excessive loading at this site. These erosions are generally about a centimetre across. Erosions are also common on the femoral side of the patello-femoral joint where they vary in cross-sectional area a good deal more than those seen under the meniscus measuring up to 4 or 5 cm across. Erosion of damaged tissue eventually may be so extensive as to completely denude the bone surface of its cartilage cover (eburnation).

The last, and less common, form of structural lesion is cracking of the cartilage. Cracks extend vertically deeply into the cartilage and microscopically have often a deep horizontal component (**3.24**).

In considering the pathogenesis of these lesions, it is important to recognize that in the early stages of OA they often affect only one of the opposed articular surfaces. This is in marked contrast to eburnation where both opposed surfaces are affected.

An increase in water content, or a decrease in proteoglycan or a combination of the two, will result in cartilage softening (chondromalacia). Chondromalacia and fibrillation generally go together, but chondromalacia may be present before fibrillation.

3.23

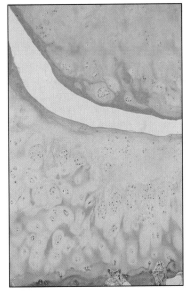

3.23 A photograph of the articular surface of the superior portion of the acetabulum. This area is characteristically fibrillated and chondromalacic, even though the femoral head cartilage is quite intact. This is believed to be due to a disuse atrophy.

3.24

3.24 A photomicrograph to demonstrate deep vertical cracks with extensive horizontal cracking (× 4).

Microscopic and biochemical changes

Injury at a cellular level may be recognizable only under a microscope. Necrosis is recognized where only the ghost outlines of chondrocytes remain. This ghosting, usually scattered but focal in distribution, is a common finding in OA (**3.25**). Less often, all chondrocytes are necrotic. Using a combination of immunohistochemical, biochemical and in-situ hybridization techniques, Von der Mark identified three types of chondrocyte in osteoarthritic cartilage (Von der Mark *et al.*, 1992). Normal chondrocytes were observed secreting Type II collagen and clusters of cells, having undergone focal dedifferentiation, were found secreting Type I and Type III collagen. In the middle and deep zones, particularly in areas with a deeply fibrillated surface, hypertrophic chondrocytes were seen producing increased amounts of Type X collagen.

The early stages of OA were marked by an increased Type I and II collagen expression, particularly in the middle zone and most prominently in the regenerated cartilage of the osteophytes.

Just as the effect of injury to the articular cartilage is reflected in the microscopic histology of both matrix and cells, so too is the effect of subsequent cartilage regeneration. In the cellular component, there is evidence of focal cellular proliferation with clumps, or clones, of chondrocytes (**3.26**). Around these clumps of proliferating chondrocytes, when the tissue is stained with toluidine blue, there is often intense metachromasia indicating increased proteoglycan content. Increased synthesis of proteoglycan by the cloned chondrocytes has been demonstrated also by an increased uptake of 35-S labelled isotope (Meachim and Collins, 1962). The degree of increased synthesis of proteoglycan, as well as collagen, appears directly proportional to the severity of the arthritis. Both may be associated with the simultaneous appearance of new chondrocytes. Analysis of changes occurring in proteoglycan composition have shown that osteoarthritic cartilage contains increased levels of keratan sulphate and a change in the ratio of different types of chondroitin sulphate. These changes could suggest that the chondrocytes revert to an immature pattern of proteoglycan secretion (Bayliss, 1992). Caterson (1992) used specific monoclonal antibodies directed against different PG epitopes detected subtle changes in chondroitin sulphate in the early stages of OA. These changes may affect the binding of growth factors to PGs and the altered proteoglycans may identify a change in the phenotypic expression of chondrocytes with the onset of disease. It is possible that identification of these subtle changes may be an aid to diagnosis and management in the future. [Less is known of the relative amounts of the different collagen types at progressive stages of the disease.]

In a damaged joint, repair of cartilage may be initiated from both or either of two possible sites (Nakata and Bullough, 1986). If it comes from damaged cartilage itself, repair takes the form of cell proliferation and synthesis of new matrix ('intrinsic' repair). If it comes from the periphery of the articulation or from the subchondral bone, the process can be considered 'extrinsic' repair. In most cases of OA, both intrinsic and extrinsic repair cartilage is found. Repair cartilage which develops from the joint margin may be seen as a cellular layer of cartilage extending over, and sometimes into, existing cartilage (**3.27**). This repair cartilage is generally much more cellular than pre-existing articular cartilage, and the chondrocytes are evenly distributed throughout the matrix. On microscopic examination, this type of repair cartilage may easily be overlooked. However, examination by polarized light clearly demonstrates discontinuity between the collagen network of the repair cartilage and those of pre-existing cartilage (**3.28**).

In those osteoarthritic joints where loss of articular cartilage has denuded underlying bone, frequently there are small pits in the bone surface from which protrude small nodules of firm white tissue (**3.29**). On microscopic examination, these nodules have the appearance of fibrocartilage (**3.30**). In some arthritic joints, these proliferating nodules arise in the marrow spaces of the subchondral bone. They may be seen to extend over the previously denuded surface to form a more-or-less continuous layer of repair tissue.

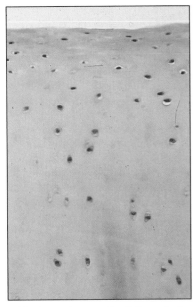

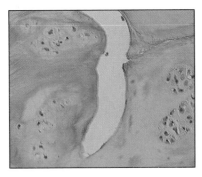

3.26 A photomicrograph to illustrate chondrocyte proliferation, or chondrone formation, in osteoarthritic cartilage (× 25).

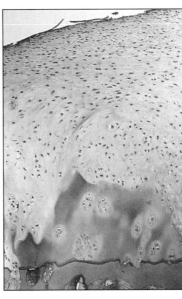

3.25 Photomicrograph of the articular cartilage from a case of OA to demonstrate focal chondrocyte necrosis (× 10).

3.27 Photomicrograph to illustrate a layer of proliferative repair cartilage overlying residual normal cartilage (× 10).

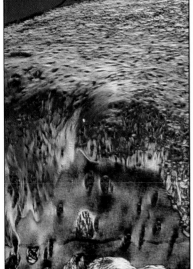

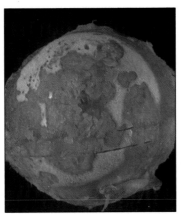

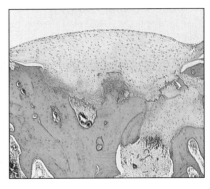

3.30 Photomicrograph of a section through one of the fibrous nodules illustrated in **3.28** shows that these nodules arise in the subchondral marrow (× 4).

3.29 A photograph of the superior articulating surface of an osteoarthritic femoral head showing multiple nodules of fibro-cartilage on the surface. In areas these nodules have a confluent pattern.

3.28 Polarized light picture of the same field as **3.27** demonstrates the discontinuity between the residual cartilage below and reparative cartilage above.

Polypeptide growth factors and cytokines

Within osteoarthritic joint tissues, there are both areas of cartilage where synthesis of new matrix is occurring and areas where net loss of the extracellular matrix occurs. It is clear that in OA, an increase in both the synthetic and degradative pathways occur followed by an uncoupling of these two pathways such that, in some areas, degradation exceeds new synthesis and vice versa. The chondrocytes are intimately involved in both of these processes and in addition to the mediators already mentioned, a range of cytokines and growth factors can affect both cartilage matrix synthesis and resorption.

The response of chondrocytes to the polypeptide growth factors (**Table 3.1**) has only recently been recognized and it is apparent that these factors play a major role both in the regulation of the synthesis of normal matrix and also in the processes involved in osteoarthritic cartilage. It is not yet clear exactly how these agents act on cartilage but many involve the presence of cell surface receptors coupled to intracellular signalling pathways. The various growth factors include insulin-like growth factor (IGF-1). This protein is structurally homologous to proinsulin sharing some 65% homology and is a similar size. IGF-1 has been found to stimulate DNA and matrix synthesis in growth plate as well as both immature and adult articular cartilage (McQuillan *et al.*, 1986). A steady state of PG synthesis is maintained by IGF-1 in adult tissue (Luyten *et al.*, 1988) and it is often more effective when it is administered with other growth factors such as EGF and b-FGF. It is thought to predominantly affect the synthesis of aggrecan whilst TGFB appears to stimulate protein synthesis in general.

Transforming growth factor-B (TGFB) is a disulphide bonded Mr 25000 polypeptide which occurs in at least five isoforms. It potentiates the stimulation of DNA synthesis achieved by b-FGF, IGF-1 and EGF rather than initiating it itself. TGFB is locally synthesized by chondrocytes and stimulates PG synthesis (Hiraki *et al.*, 1988). It is also known to stimulate the production of the metalloproteinase inhibitor TIMP by connective tissue cells (Wright *et al.*, 1991), as well as other proteinase inhibitors, suggesting that it may prevent cartilage destruction by both stimulating synthesis and blocking breakdown pathways. Addition of TGFB to cartilage stimulated to resorb with interleukin-1 (IL-1) prevents the release of proteoglycan fragments from the tissue (Andrews *et al.*, 1989).

Platelet derived growth factor (PDGF) is a major growth material for connective tissue cells and consists of a dimer of two disulphide bonded polypeptide chains. PDGF has a mitogenic effect on chondrocytes (Howes *et al.*, 1988) but its role in the normal joint is unclear although it could be involved in repair mechanisms of osteoarthritic cartilage.

Fibroblast growth factor FGF, previously described as cartilage growth factor, acts in connective tissues as a powerful mitogen and stimulates DNA synthesis in adult articular chondrocytes in culture (Osbourne *et al.*, 1989). It is likely that this factor is involved in stimulating repair within cartilage.

These growth factors are unlikely to act on their own and many are known to act synergistically in promoting matrix synthesis. The properties of growth factors known to affect cartilage are shown in **Table 3.1**. Some such as TGFB and IGF can be synthesized within the cartilage by chondrocytes and these two growth factors are known to antagonize the effects of the proinflammatory cytokines IL-1 and tumor necrosis factor (TNF) (Tyler *et al.*, 1992).

Table 3.1 Growth factors known to affect cartilage metabolism.

Growth Factor	Major function in cartilage
TGFβ	Chondrocyte proliferation promotes formation of matrix, modulates IL–1 effects, promotes synthesis of proteinase inhibitors.
PDGF	Proliferation of chondrocytes.
bFGF	Proliferation and differentiation of chondrocytes, proteinase production.
IGF–1	Proliferation of chondrocytes, GAG synthesis.
IL–1	Induction of proteinases, PGE2 and other cytokines, inhibition of GAG synthesis.
TNFα	Similar catabolic effects as IL–1.
IL–6	Proteinase inhibitor production, proliferation of chondrocytes.

The cytokines IL-1 and TNF when added to cartilage both stimulate the degradation of the matrix and the release of proteoglycan fragments within 12-24 hours. At the same time, the synthesis of matrix components is also down regulated. IL-1 is more potent than TNF although both agents are more potent if added together. The release of collagen fragments occurs much later, often after ten days in culture, and is not so reproducible. Consequently, the vast majority of work has concentrated on the release of proteoglycan fragments even though it is widely accepted that irreversible damage to cartilage structure does not occur until the collagen framework has been removed. It is not known how proteoglycan and collagen turnover is increased after treatment with IL-1 and TNF but these cytokines both stimulate the production of large amounts of stromelysin and collagenase, two proteinases (see below) known to be able to degrade proteoglycan and collagen respectively. When TGFB is added to cartilage in addition to IL-1, it blocks the release of PG fragments in a dose dependent fashion. This could be accomplished by reversing the effect that IL-1 has in preventing PG synthesis or it could stimulate the production of TIMP by chondrocytes thus preventing cartilage degradation (**3.31**).

Retinoic acid, retinol and lipopolysaccharide can also initiate the release of proteoglycan fragments from cartilage. Interestingly, retinoic acid is known to downregulate the metalloproteinases stromelysin and collagenase as well as upregulate their inhibitor, tissue inhibitor of metalloproteinases (TIMP) (Wright *et al.*, 1991) and this apparent contradiction in the actions of retinoic acid and IL-1 on cartilage has not as yet been adequately explained.

3.31

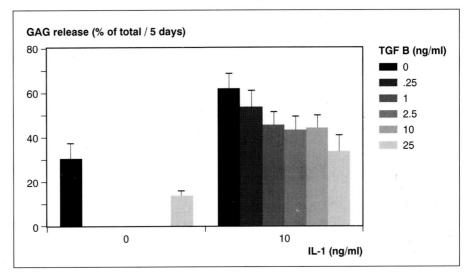

3.31. Effect of TGFB on the release of PG fragments from cartilage stimulated with IL-1. Porcine articular cartilage was cultured for three days in the presence or absence of IL-1. IL-1 stimulated the relase of PG fragments. However, in the presence of increasing concentrations of TGFB (0—25ng/ml), a dose dependent inhibition of release was observed in both IL-1 stimulated and control cartilage. TGFB is known to stimulate the release of TIMP the metalloproteinase inhibitor and increase the synthesis of matrix components.

Proteinases involved in matrix turnover

Enzymes that can degrade proteins by cleaving at specific points along the polypeptide chain are divided into four main groups according to the amino acid or chemical group that occurs at the active site. These groups consist of the cysteine and aspartate proteinases which act at an acid pH and are thought to be responsible for intracellular digestion of proteins. The serine and metalloproteinases act at neutral pH and are responsible in general for extracellular turnover of protein. The proteinases that are known to be able to breakdown collagen and proteoglycan are listed in **Table 3.2.** Proteinases from all the above classes are included with a list of known inhibitors and the substrates that are known to be cleaved. It is interesting to note that the enzymes that act at neutral pH have a limited action on cross-linked insoluble collagen.

In the 1950s, collagen was regarded as a protein

that was totally resistant to proteolytic attack within the body as only bacterial enzymes were known to be able to break down this protein. In 1962, Gross and Lapierre discovered an enzyme capable of specifically cleaving collagen in the resorbing tail of a tadpole. They named this enzyme collagenase and showed that it cleaved collagen at one point through all three α chains three quarters of the way from the N-terminal end. Since this time, a whole family of potent enzymes have been described that between them can destroy all the protein components of the extracellular matrix. These enzymes, called the matrix metalloproteinases (MMPs) are made up of common building blocks as shown in **3.32** and fall into three main groups which differ in size, called the stromelysins, gelatinases and collagenases (Woessner, 1991). The catalytic mechanism depends on zinc at the active centre and each enzyme is secreted with a propeptide attached which has to be removed before matrix can be degraded. This activation involves other proteinases possible plasmin generated by plasminogen activator, other members of the MMP family or membrane bound proteinases. The main substrates of the enzyme are shown in **Table 3.3**. All the enzymes are inhibited by the tissue inhibitor of metalloproteinases (TIMP) (Cawston et al., 1981) and all connective tissues contain members of the TIMP family. TIMP is a glycoprotein of Mr 28000 containing 184 amino acids held together by six disulphide bridges to form two main domains. The mechanism of inhibition is not known but TIMP is very similar in structure to a second protein of 194 amino acids recently named

TIMP-2 (Stetler-Stevenson et al., 1989). Both proteins are very stable and bind very tightly to the active forms of all the members of the MMP family in a 1:1 ratio.

Because these enzymes are so potent, they must be carefully controlled. The synthesis and secretion of the collagenases and stromelysins are stimulated by pro-inflammatory cytokines such as IL-1 and TNF. The collagenases degrade the fibrillar collagens and the stromelysins can degrade PGs and some basement membrane components. However, once activated, the enzymes can be blocked if sufficient available TIMP is present. This inhibitor blocks the activity of all the active forms of the enzymes by binding very tightly to form a 1:1 complex (Cawston et al., 1983). Consequently, if TIMP levels exceed those of active enzyme then connective tissue turnover is stopped. **3.33** illustrates the main components involved in these processes, however, it is likely that these events are tightly controlled and take place close to the cell membrane.

The involvement of these proteinases in the normal turnover of connective tissue matrix that takes place is well established. In addition, these enzymes have been extracted from (Dean, 1989) and localized in osteoarthritic cartilage using a number of different techniques (Brinkerhoff, 1991).

Much interest has been shown in the role of stromelysin in the degradation of PG's released into OA synovial fluid and from cartilage in organ culture systems. Stromelysin can readily degrade PG's, and IL-1 stimulates its synthesis and secretion, thus

Table 3.2 Proteinases involved in the turnover of connective tissue matrix. The ability of different cysteine, aspartic, serine and metalloproteinases to degrade collagen and proteoglycan is tabulated with the known inhibitors of each enzyme and the pH range at which it can act.

Proteinase	Class	Inhibitors	pH range	Core protein	Insoluble helical collagen	Solubilized helical collagen
Cathepsin B	Cys	Cystatins α2M		Yes	Yes	Yes
Cathepsin L	Cys	Cystatins α2M	3–5.5	Yes	Yes	Yes
Cathepsin H	Cys	Cystatins α2M		?	Yes	Yes
Cathepsin D	Asp	α2M	4–6	Yes	No	No
Plasmin	Ser	α2M, α1AC, α1PI		Yes	No	No
Elastase	Ser	α2M, α1AC, α1PI	6–9	Yes	No	No
Cathepsin G	Ser	α2M, α1AC, α1PI		Yes	No	No
Stromelysin	Metallo	TIMP,TIMP-2,α2M	4–5.9	Yes	No	No
Collagenase	Metallo	TIMP,TIMP-2,α2M	7–8	No	Limited	Yes
Gelatinase	Metallo	TIMP,TIMP-2,α2M	7–8	?	No	No

promoting cartilage resorption. In addition, stromelysin is found in raised amounts of OA cartilage and it was assumed that stromelysin was responsible for the cleavage of proteoglycan. However, recent data suggests that a further enzyme may be involved. It is known that the cleavage of aggrecan in IL-1 stimulated and osteoarthritic cartilage occurs between the G1 and G2 domains.

Although it is known that stromelysins cleave in this region, sequence analysis of PG fragments in synovial fluids (Sandy *et al.*, 1992) and in released fragments from organ culture experiments (Flannery, 1992) reveal a different cleavage point from that expected if stromelysin was responsible for cutting the polypeptide chain. This cleavage is thought to be made by an unidentified enzyme named aggrecanase although it has yet to be purified and characterized. It is likely that the enzyme pathways responsible for cartilage destruction involve the metalloproteinases since the release of proteoglycan and collagen from resorbing cartilage in experimental systems can be prevented with highly specific low molecular weight synthetic inhibitors (Andrews, Plumpton *et al.*, 1992). **3.34** illustrates the effect of adding increasing amounts of such an inhibitor to pig articular cartilage fragments incubated with IL-1 for three days. The release of PG fragments was completely prevented at the highest concentration of inhibitor. It is likely that such inhibitors could be of therapeutic benefit in preventing the destruction of cartilage in OA.

Recent work has also suggested that inhibitors of cysteine proteinases, that are targeted to cross cell membranes and so enter cells, can also block cartilage resorption (Buttle *et al.*, 1992). This suggests that multiple pathways are involved and that these depend on other classes of proteinases and that a mixture of extracellular and intracellular breakdown of cartilage matrix components occurs.

Most recent work has focussed on PG breakdown in cartilage resorption to the exclusion of other matrix components. It is known that the turnover of PG is both rapid and reversible as compared with collagen. Injection of IL-1 into rabbits knee joints causes a rapid loss of PG which is rapidly replaced by new synthesis (Page-Thomas, 1991). The gross loss of the collagen fibrillar network from cartilage is irreversible in the sense that any attempt at repair is unlikely to lead to restoration of normal cartilage matrix structure. In future, greater attention should be paid to targetting collagenase as a valid therapeutic objective in OA.

Table 3.3 Matrix metalloproteinases and the connective tissue components that they can digest. The different combinations of the domain structures of the matrix metalloproteinases alters their substrate specificity. The different substrates digested by each proteinase is listed in the table.

Enzyme	Matrix substrate
Interstitial collagenase	Collagen types I, II, III, VII, X
MMP–1	Gelatin
Neutrophil collagenase	Collagen types I, II, III
MMP–8	
72-kd gelatinase	Gelatin types I, II, III, elastin
MMP–2	Collagen types IV, V, VII, X, fibronectin
92-kd gelatinase	Gelatins I, V
MMP–9	Collagen types IV, V
Stromelysin–1	Proteoglycan, fibronectin, laminin
MMP–3	Gelatin types I, III, IV, V
	Collagen types III, IV, V, IX
	Procollagen propeptides, activates procollagenase
Stromelysin–2	Gelatin types I, III, IV, V
MMP–10	Weak on collagen types III, IV, V fibronectin, activates procollagenase
Matrilysin	Gelatin types I, III, IV, V
MMP–7	activates procollagenase proteoglycan, fibronectin

3.32

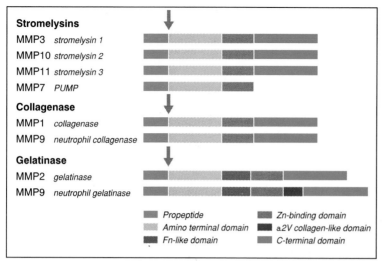

3.32 The molecular structure of the matrix metalloproteinases. The metalloproteinases are divided into three main groups: the stromelysins, the collagenases and the gelatinases, but are closely related in that they all contain related domains. All proteinases contain a propeptide domain, N-terminal domain and zinc binding domain, but differ in the presence of a C-terminal domain and the gelatinases are characterized by the addition of extra sequences of protein.

3.33

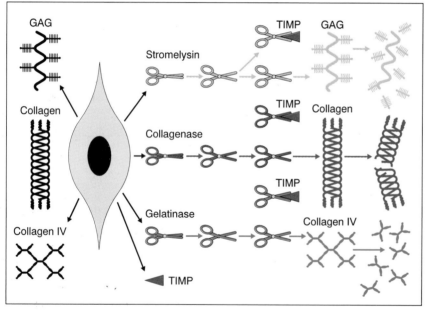

3.33 Control of the matrix metalloproteinases after leaving the cell. Connective tissue cells in addition to synthesizing matrix components also make a family of proteinases that can chop up all the different components of connective tissue. The enzymes are produced in an inactive form which require activation. This takes place after the removal of a small sequence of polypeptide chain by proteolytic attack. The cells also produce a specific inhibitor called TIMP that can bind to the active forms of the enzyme and prevent them from working. If excess TIMP is present, then no breakdown of connective tissue occurs. The metalloproteinases are switched on by IL-1 and TNF whilst TIMP is switched on by TGFB.

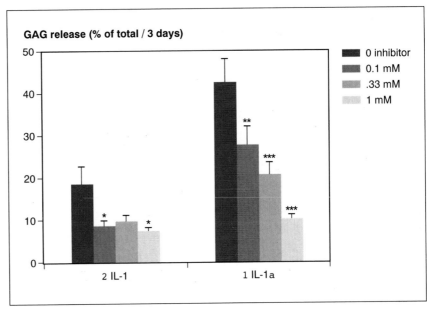

GAG release (% of total / 3 days)

Legend:
- 0 inhibitor
- 0.1 mM
- .33 mM
- 1 mM

3.34 The release of PG fragments from IL1-treated cartilage is prevented by low Mr synthetic inhibitors of metalloproteinases.

Injury and repair of bone

Osteoarthritis is a disease that also profoundly affects the underlying bone and the structures around the joint. As the articular cartilage is eroded from the articular surface, the underlying bone becomes polished or eburnated (**3.35**), and is subjected to increasingly localized overloading. In subarticular bone, which has been so denuded, there is proliferation of osteoblasts and formation of new bone. This new bone formation can be seen microscopically to occur both on the surfaces of existing intact trabeculae, and as a result of microfractures. In radiographs of arthritic joints, new bone production results in increased density or sclerosis. Radiologically, it is particularly evident beneath joint surfaces where the joint space, i.e. the cartilage, has largely disappeared. Studies of the localization of alkaline and acid phosphatase (markers of osteoblastic and osteoclastic activity) in osteoarthritic femoral heads, have shown that there is an increase in subchondral bone enzyme activity proportionate to the severity of cartilaginous change (Christensen, 1985). The highest enzyme levels being found in denuded weightbearing areas of bone and in the osteophytes. The lowest enzyme levels were found in non-weightbearing subchondral bone and more centrally within the femoral head. A further result of increased local stress is that the exposed surface bone is likely to undergo focal pressure necrosis (**3.36**). This superficial necrosis has to be distinguished from 'primary' osteonecrosis, which may of its own accord lead to secondary OA. In clinical practice a differentiation between primary and secondary disease may be difficult especially in the late stages of primary osteonecrosis (Franchi and Bullough, 1992).

Subarticular cysts in cases of OA are seen only where the overlying cartilage is absent. Such cysts are common and are thought to be the result of transmission of intra-articular pressure through defects in the articulating bony surface into the marrow spaces of the subchondral bone. The cysts increase in size until the pressure within them is equal to the intra-articular pressure (Landells, 1953). Cysts may also occur because of focal tissue necrosis (Rhaney and Lamb, 1955).

In the late stages of OA, the articular surface of the damaged joint may become covered by regenerative cartilage; the pressure on the joint surface is again more equitably distributed, and cysts frequently regress, and even disappear.

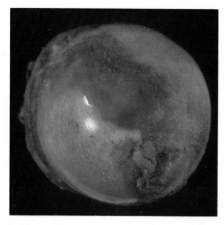

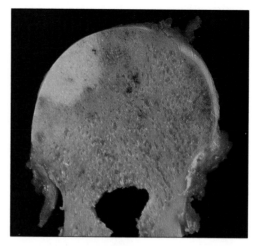

3.35 A photograph of a femoral head removed from a patient with OA, demonstrating loss of cartilage from the superior and lateral articular surface with exposure of the underlying bone which has a polished (eburnated) appearance.

3.36 A photograph of a coronal section through an osteoarthritic femoral head showing some superficial bone necrosis; recognized by the dull yellowish white appearance of the necrotic bone surrounded by a slightly darker hyperemic border. Superficial necrosis of this type is common in OA and should be distinguished from primary segmental avascular necrosis.

Loose Bodies

Separated fragments of bone and cartilage from a damaged joint surface may become incorporated into the synovial membrane, and digested. On the other hand, they may form loose bodies in the joint cavity. Under certain circumstances, proliferation of the cartilage cells occurs on the surface of these loose bodies and consequently they grow in size. As they grow, their centres become necrotic and calcified. In histologic sections, it is possible to visualize periodic extension of this central calcification, in the form of concentric rings increasing in number as the loose body grows larger. Sometimes the bodies may reattach to the synovial membrane, in which case they become invaded by blood vessels and re-ossified.

In most cases of OA, there is some degree of loose body formation. Occasionally, if the loose bodies are numerous, they need to be distinguished from those which occur in primary synovial chondromatosis (Villacin *et al.*, 1979).

Ligaments

In the ligamentous and capsular tissue around an arthritic joint, microscopic evidence of both lacerations and of repair by scar tissue are common findings. Whether these might have preceded the arthritis process or whether they are a consequence of it cannot be determined by microscopic examination. Little work has been initiated on tendon and ligament diseases and little is known about these tissues. Tendon cells can be recovered from normal tendon and can product Type I collagen as well as enzymes and inhibitors involved in matrix turnover (Chard, 1987), but is not known how these tissues are affected in OA.

Injury of the synovial membrane

Injury and breakdown of cartilage and bone result in increased amounts of breakdown product and particulate debris within the joint cavity. The debris is removed from the synovial fluid by phagocytic cells (the 'A' cells) of the synovial membrane. In consequence of overactivity, the membrane becomes both hypertrophic and hyperplastic. The breakdown products of cartilage and bone matrix evoke an inflammatory response (3.37) and for this reason, some degree of chronic inflammation is to be expected in the synovial membrane of the arthritic joints, even when the injury has been purely a mechanical one. Inflammation is especially prominent where there has been rapid breakdown of the articular components as

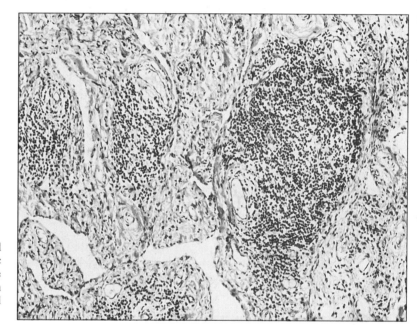

3.37

3.37 A photomicrograph of synovial tissue obtained from an osteoarthritic joint. There is hyperplasia of the synovial lining cells together with an infiltration of both lymphocytes and plasma cells (× 4).

evidenced by the presence in the synovium of bone and cartilage detritus.

Histological studies have shown that there may be a similarity between the degree of inflammatory response, as seen in some cases of severe osteoarthritis, and in rheumatoid arthritis (Ito and Bullough, 1979). However, in OA, the synovial inflammation is probably the result of cartilage breakdown.

Extension of the hyperplastic synovium on to the articular surface of the joint, i.e. a pannus, is a common finding even in OA, particularly the hip. However, the extent and the aggressiveness of this pannus with respect to underlying cartilage destruction is much less marked in OA than that seen in patients suffering from rheumatoid arthritis (3.38).

Under normal conditions, the synovial membrane is responsible for the nutrition of articular cartilage. In this regard, it might be expected that the chronically inflamed and scarred synovial membrane of OA may function less well than normal. Disturbance in synovial nutrient function may well contribute to the chronicity of the arthritic process. The hypertrophied and hyperplastic synovium is likely to be itself damaged as the increased amount of synovial tissue extends into the joint cavity and it is traumatized and evidence of chronic bleeding in the form of hemosiderin pigment is a common finding.

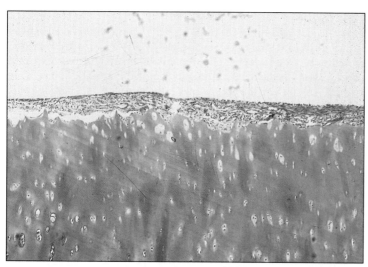

3.38 A photomicrograph to demonstrate a fibrous pannus injury on the articular surface of the cartilage in a case of OA of the hip. Although in rheumatoid arthritis, the pannus is likely to be more extensive and more destructive, pannus is not uncommon in cases of OA especially in the hip joint (× 4).

Synovial fluid in an injured joint

Normal synovial fluid, a dialysate of plasma, to which hyaluronic acid produced by 'B' cells of the synovial lining is added, is viscous, pale yellow and clear. The volume, even in large joints, is small. Examination of synovial fluid is extremely helpful in the diagnosis of arthritis, both in determining the cause and the stage of the disease. Whatever the cause of arthritis, the synovial fluid will be altered.

In inflammatory arthritis, there is an increased volume of synovial fluid and the amount of hyaluronic acid is markedly diminished. This leads to a typical decrease in viscosity. However, in degenerate forms of arthritis the amount of hyaluronic acid is increased.

This produces an extremely viscous fluid. There is often also an increase in volume although not to the same degree as seen in inflammatory arthritis.

Blood chemistry investigations, cell counts and various immune reaction tests may help to indicate the specific nature of the arthritis in question. Recent studies have suggested that analysis of degraded matrix components released into the synovial fluid may indicate the degree of cartilage destruction and so act as disease markers. The use of synovial fluid markers is discussed in Chapters 6 and 10.

Pathogenesis of OA

A number of autopsy studies have demonstrated the incidence of OA in various joints as well as its progression from mild to severe disease (Collins, 1938; Heine, 1926). Generally, attempts to grade the disease have been based solely on morphologic findings but more recently, attempts at grading have included histochemical and biochemical parameters as well (Mankin *et al.*, 1971).

The availability of a large volume of tissue specimens from hip replacement arthroplasty now makes it possible to gain further insights into the natural history of OA of the hip. In 1980, we published our observations on the natural history, based upon a study of case histories, radiographs and tissue specimens from 234 operated hips in 183 patients (Macys *et al.*, 1980). All of these patients were considered both clinically and morphologically, to have primary (senile or idiopathic) OA of the hip.

One of the problems with most classifications of the radiographic changes in OA is that they tend to miss the dynamic progressive nature of the disease which involves both mechanical wear, cell injury and repair. In our study, we attempted to stage the disease on the basis of horizontal comparisons of radiographs in different patients' hips but also in longitudinal studies of serial hip radiographs of the same patient.

We defined Stage I disease as cartilage narrowing or absence with preservation of the subchondral bone contours of the femoral head and of the acetabulum. In this early stage of the disease, migration of the femoral head had not occurred beyond the distance of the loss of the cartilage space (**3.39**).

Radiographic Stage II was defined as complete absence of the superior joint space with incomplete or complete loss of the subchondral bone contour. In this stage, bone loss may be marked and subchondral sclerosis and cystic changes in the bone are prominent. Migration of the joint in most cases superiorly and laterally has also occurred relative to the bone loss (**3.40**).

The final stage, radiographic Stage III, is characterized by some reappearance of the joint space

3.39

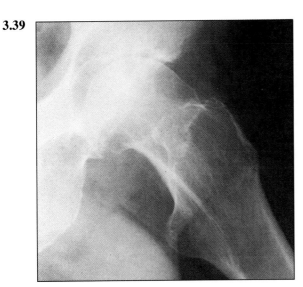

3.39 Radiograph to demonstrate Stage I OA (see text).

3.40

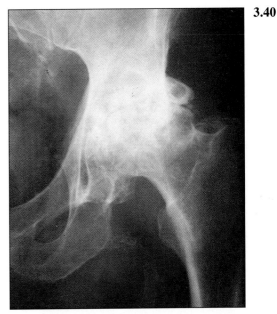

3.40 Radiograph to demonstrate Stage II OA (see text).

after maximal bone loss and migration have occurred. The bony contours again become relatively well-defined. Sclerosis has diminished and cysts have become indistinct (**3.41**). The radiologic staging corresponded well to the duration of symptoms.

A number of correlations between this system of radiographic staging and the pathological appearances of the resected specimens could be made. The most striking of these correlations were that reparative cartilage was much more prominent in radiographic Stage III than it was in Stage I. Subchondral cysts were most prevalent in Stage II and tended to decrease in number in Stage III. It was also noted that cysts appeared earlier and more commonly on the acetabular side of the joint than on the femoral side of the joint indicating perhaps that degeneration on the acetabular side of the joint precedes that on the femoral side.

That some cases of OA improve spontaneously both symptomatically and radiographically, has been documented in several clinical studies (Pearson and Riddell, 1962; Perry *et al.*, 1972; Seifert *et al.*, 1969). In a series of 91 hips which were not operated on and which were followed for ten years, Danielson found that 2/3 reported a decrease in pain and that radiographic follow-up showed a real or apparent regression of the arthritic changes in 7% of the cases (Danielsson, 1964). A number of other authors have reported cases of OA in which radiographic recovery of the joint space occurred after an average of about 10 years of symptomatic disease. Interestingly, similar radiological and histological changes have been described following surgical osteotomy (Storey and Landells, 1971).

Remodelling of bone occurs early in OA. It results in subchondral bone thickening as well as the formation of marginal osteophytes. The degree of remodelling through osteophyte formation can be considerable but the presence of osteophytes in the knee and hip by no means always heralds development of progressive symptomatic OA. Radiographic studies have shown that 2/3 of the knees which have evidence of osteophyte formation, even when followed up for as long as 17 years, do not develop other degenerative changes (Lawrence *et al.*, 1966).

3.41

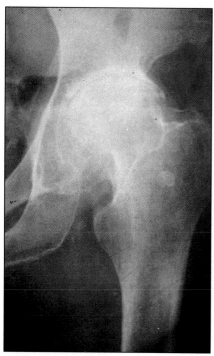

3. 41 A clinical radiograph of a patient with advanced OA followed without treatment for 9 years (see text).

Aetiology

The aetiology of arthritis can be stated in general terms to be any condition which will change the shape of the articulating surface, change the support or alter the tissue matrices. For example, a fracture through an articular surface will alter the geometry of a joint.

Another condition which leads to altered joint shape is excessive or altered modeling at the bone cartilage interface such as occurs (dramatically) in Paget's disease (**3.42**) and various endocrinopathies, especially acromegaly (Johanson, 1985). Ligament injury is a well-recognized antecedent of OA (e.g. meniscal and anterior cruciate injury in the knee). Surgical removal of a meniscus will also significantly affect load distribution and stability in the knee and may of itself eventually contribute to the development of OA. If, as happens in ochronosis, the cartilage is rendered stiffer and more brittle, with use it begins to disintegrate and arthritis ensues.

As has already been emphasized, the joints which develop OA are those which show evidence of cartilage degeneration in early adulthood. Contrary to previously expressed views that these areas are degenerate because of excessive loading, we and others have taken the view that these areas are degenerate because of underuse rather than overuse (Harrison *et al.*, 1953). It is possible that with alterations in joint modeling, as for example, occurs with various endocrinopathies and as a normal result of ageing, these areas of "disuse change" have a contributory role in accelerating cartilage breakdown in turn leading to the development of clinical OA.

Thus alterations in shape, ligament stability and tissue properties can result in arthritis. However, OA is a disease of multiple etiologies and looking for a single cause of OA is fruitless. Dysfunction may begin in any of the structures that make up the joint, but by the time the disease comes to the attention of a clinician, most structures of the joint are involved. Because of this overall involvement, it is generally impossible for the pathologist to determine the etiology in any particular case of arthritis, especially in the later stages of the disease.

3.42

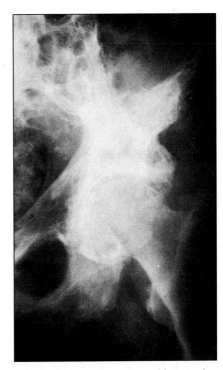

3.42 Radiograph of a patient with extensive Paget's disease of the pelvis. There is a marked alteration in the shape of the acetabulum with loss of joint space. Paget's disease will sometimes present with joint pain.

References and further reading

Ali, S.Y., Anderson, H.C., Sajdera, S.W. (1971) Enzymatic and electromicroscopic analysis of extracellular matrix vesicles associated with calcification in cartilage. *Biochem. J.*, **122**, 56.

Anderson, H.C. (1980) Calcification processes. *Pathol. Ann.*, **15** (2), 45–75.

Andrews, H.J., Edwards, T.A., Cawston, T.E., Hazleman, B.L. (1989) TGFB causes partial inhibition of IL-1 stimulated cartilage degradation in vitro. *Biochem. Biophys. Res. Comm.*, **162**, 144–150.

Andrews, H.J., Plumpton, T.A., Harper, G.P., Cawston, T.E. (1992) A synthetic peptide inhibitor but not TIMP prevents the breakdown of PG within articular cartilage in vitro. *Agents and Actions*, **37**, 147–154.

Bayliss, M.T. (1992) Metabolism of animal and human OA cartilage. In Kuettner, K., *et al.* (Eds). *Articular cartilage and osteoarthritis*. Raven Press, New York, 487–500.

Bennett, G.A., Waine, H., Bauer, W. (1942) Changes in the knee joint at various ages, with particular reference to the nature and development of degenerative joint disease. New York, The Commonwealth Fund.

Bianco, P., Fisher, L.W., Young, M.F., Termine, J.D., Robey, P.G. (1990) Expression and localization of two small proteoglycans biglycan and decorin in developing skeletal and non-skeletal tissue. *J. Histochem. Cytochem.*, **38**, 1549–1563.

Bjelle, A. (1975) Content and composition of glycosaminoglycans in human knee joint cartilage. *Connect Tissue Res.*, **3**: 141–147.

Blumenthal, N.C., Posner, A.S., Silverman, L.D., Rosenberg, L.C. (1979) The effect of proteoglycans on in vitro hydroxyapatite formation. *Calcif. Tissue Int.*, **27**, 75–82.

Blumenthal. N.C., Betts, F, Posner, A.S. (1977) Stabilization of amorphous calcium phosphate by Mg and ATP. *Calcif. Tissue Int.*, **23**, 245–250.

Boskey, A.L. (1978) The role of $Ca-PL-PO_4$ complexes in tissue mineralization. *Metab. Bone Dis.*, **1**, 137–148.

Boskey, A.L. (1979) Models of matrix vesicle calcification. *Inorg. Perspect. Biol. Med.*, **2**, 51–54.

Boskey, A.L., Bullough, P.G., Dmitrovsky, E. (1980) The biochemistry of the mineralization front. *Metab. Bone Dis. Rel. Res.*, **2S**: 61–67.

Boyan-Salyers, B.D. (1980) Proteolipid and calcification of cartilage. *Trans. Orthop. Res. Soc.*, **5**, 9–13.

Brinckerhoff, C.E. (1991) Joint destruction in arthritis. MMPs in the spotlight. A&R, **34**, 1073–1075.

Bullough, P.G., Goodfellow, J., O'Connor, J.J. (1973) The relationship between degenerative changes and load bearing in the human hip. *J. Bone Joint Surg.* (Br.), **55**, 746–758.

Bullough, P.G., Goodfellow, J.W. (1968) The significance of the fine structure of articular cartilage. *J. Bone Joint Surg., (Br.)*, **50** (4), 852–857.

Bullough, P.G., Jagannath, A., (1983) The morphology of the calcification front in articular cartilage. *J. Bone Joint Surg. (Br.)*, **65**, 72–78.

Bullough, P.G., Munuera, L., Murphy, J., Weinstein, A. (1970) The strength of the menisci of the knee as it relates to their fine structure. *J. Bone Joint Surg. (Br.)* **52**, 564–570.

Bullough, P.G., Walker, P.S., (1977) The distribution of load through the knee joint and its possible significance to the observed patterns of articular cartilage cartilage breakdown. *Bull. Hosp. Joint Dis. Orthop. Inst.* **37**, 110–123.

Bullough, P.G., Yawitz, P.S., Tafra, L., *et al.* (1985) Topographical variations in the morphology and biochemistry of adult canine tibial plateau articular cartilage. *J. Orthop. Res.*, **3**, 1–16.

Buttle, D.J., Saklatval, J., Tamai, M., Barrett, A.J. (1992) Inhibition of IL-1 stimulated cartilage proteoglycan degradation by a lipophilic inactivator of cysteine endopeptidases. *Biochem. J.*, **281**, 175–177.

Byers, P.D., Contepomi, C.A., Farkas, T.A. (1970) A post-mortem study of the hip joint. *Ann. Rheum. Dis.*, **29**, 15.

Caterson, B., Hughes, C.E., Johnstone, B., Mort, J.S. (1992) Immunological markers of cartilage proteoglycan metabolism in animal and human OA. In Kuettner, K., *et al.* (Eds). *Articular cartilage and osteoarthritis*. Raven Press, New York, 415–428.

Caterson, B., Lowther, D.A. (1978) Changes in the metabolism of the proteoglycans from sheep articular cartilage in response to mechanical stress. *Biochim. Biophys. Acta.*, **540**, 412–422.

Cawston, T.E., Galloway, W.A., Mercer, E., Murphy, G., Reynolds, J.J. (1981) *Biochem. J.*, **195**, 159–165.

Cawston, T.E., Murphy, G., Mercer, E., Galloway, W.A., Hazleman, B.L., Reynolds, J.J. (1983) The interaction of purified rabbit bone collagenase with purified rabbit bone meyalloproteinase inhibitor. *Biochem. J.*, **211.**, 313–318.

Chard, M.D., Wright, J.K., Hazleman, B.L. (1987) Isolation and growth characteristics of adult human tendon fibroblasts. *Ann. Rheum. Dis.*, **46**, 385–390.

Christensen, S.B. (1985) Osteoarthrosis: changes in bone, cartilage and synovial membrane in relation to bone scintigraphy. *Acta Orthop. Scan. Suppl.*, **214** (56), 1–43.

Collins, D.H. (1938) The pathology of osteoarthritis. *Br. J. Rheumatism*, **14**, 253.

Danielsson, L.G. (1964) Incidence and prognosis of coxarthrosis. *Acta Orthop. Scand. Suppl.*, **66**: 1–114.

Dean, D.D., Martel-Pelletier, J., Martel-Pelletier, J.P., Howell, D.S. and Woessner, J. (1989) MMP & TIMP imbalance in human osteoarthritic cartilage. *J. Clin. Invest.*, **84**, 678–685.

DeWitt, M.T., Handley, C.J., Oakes, B.W., Lowther, D.A. (1984) In vitro response of chondrocytes to mechanical loading. The effect of short term mechanical tension. *Connect. Tissue Res.*, **12**, 97–109.

Eyre, D.R., Wu, J.J., Woods, P. (1992) Cartilage-specific collagens–structural studies. In Kuettner, K., *et al.* (Eds) *Articular cartilage and osteoarthritis*. Raven Press, New York.

Felix, R., Fleisch, H. (1976) Pyrophosphatase and ATPase of isolated cartilage matrix vesicles. *Calcif. Tissue Int.*, **22**: 1–7.

Flannery, C.R., Lark, M.W., and Sandy, J.D. (1992) Identification of a stromelysin cleavage site within the interglobular domain of human aggrecan. *J. Biol. Chem.*, **267**, 1008–1014.

Fortuna, R., Anderson, H.C., Carty, R.P., Sajdera, S.W.

(1979) Enzymatic characterization of the chondrocytic alkaline phosphatase isolated from bovine fetal epiphyseal cartilage. *Biochim. Biophys. Acta.*, **570**, 291–302.

Franchi, A., Bullough, P.G (1992) Secondary avascular necrosis in coxarthrosis; a morphologic study. *J. Rheumatol.*, **19**, 1263–1268.

Goodfellow, J.W., Bullough, P.G. (1967) The pattern of ageing of the articular cartilage of the elbow joint. *J. Bone Joint Surg. (Br.)*, **49**, 175–181.

Gross, J., Lapiere, C.M. (1962) Collagenolytic activity in amphibian tissues: a tissue culture assay. *Proc. Natl. Acad. Sci. USA*, **54**, 1197–1204.

Hammond, B.T., Charnley, J. (1967) The sphericity of the femoral head. *J. Med. Biol. Eng.*, **5**, 445.

Harrison, M.H.M., Schajowicz, F., Trueta, J. (1953) Osteoarthritis of the hip: a study of the nature and evolution of the disease. *J. Bone Joint Surg. (Br.)*, **35**, 598.

Hascall, V.C. (1988) Proteoglycans: the chondroitin sulphate keratan sulphate proteoglycan of cartilage. *ISI Atlas of Science.* Biochemistry. 189–198.

Heine, J (1926). Uber die Arthritis deformans. *Virchows Arch.*, **260,** 521–663.

Heinegard, D.K., Pimental, E.R. (1992) Cartilage matrix proteins. In Kuettner, K. *et al.* (Eds) *Articular cartilage and osteoarthritis.* Raven Press, New York, 95–117.

Hiraki, Y., Inoue, H., Hirai, R., Kato, Y., Suzuki, F (1988) Effect of TGFB on cell proliferation and GAG synthesis by rabbit growth plate chondrocytes in culture. *Biochem. Biophys. Acta.*, **969**, 91–99.

Houston, J.P., McGuire, M.K.B., Meats, J.E., Ebsworth, N.M., Russell, R.G.G., Crawford, A., MacNeil, S. (1982) Adenylate cyclase of human articular chondrocytes. *Biochem. J.*, **208**, 35–42.

Howes, R., Bowness, J.M., Grotendorst, G.R., Martin, G.R., Reddi, A.H. (1988) PDFG enhances demineralized bone matrix-induced cartilage and bone formation. *Calcif. Tiss. Int.*, **42**, 34–38.

Hunter, W. (1743) Of the structure and diseases of articulating cartilages. *Phil. Trans.*, 267–271.

Ito. S., Bullough, P.G, (1979) Synovial and osseous inflammation in degenerative joint disease and rheumatoid arthritis of the hip. Histometric study. *Proceedings of the 25th Annual ORS*, 199.

Johansen, N.A. (1985) Endocrine arthropathies. *Clin. Rheum. Dis.* II (2), 297–323.

Johnson, L.C. (1964) Morphologic analysis in pathology: the kinetics of disease and general biology of bone. In Frost, H.M. (Ed.), *Bone biodynamics.* Little, Brown and Company, Boston, 543–654.

Jones, I.L., Klamfeldt, A., Sandstrom, T. (1982) The effect of continuous mechanical pressure upon the turnover of articular cartilage proteoglycans in vitro. *Clin. Orthop.*, **165**, 283–289.

Kempson, G.E., Muir, H., Swanson, A., Freeman, M.A.R. (1970) Correlates between stiffness and the chemical constituents of cartilage of the human femoral head. *Biochim. Biophys. Acta.*, **215**, 70–77.

Kosher, R.A., Savage, M.P. (1980) Studies on the possible role of cyclic AMP in limb morphogenesis and differentiation. *J. Embryol. Exp. Morphol.*, **56**, 91–105.

Landells, J.W. (1953) The bone cysts of osteoarthritis. *J. Bone Joint Surg., (Br.)*, **35**, 643.

Lane, L.B., Villacin, A.B., Bullough, P.G. (1977) The vascularity and remodelling of subchondral bone and calcified cartilage in adult human femoral and humeral heads. An age-and-stress-related phenomenon. *J. Bone Joint Surg.(Br.)*, **59**, 272–278.

Lawrence, J.S., Brenner, J.M., Bier, F. (1966) Osteoarthrosis: Prevalence in population and relationship between symptoms and X-ray changes. *Ann. Rheum. Dis.*, **25**, 1–24.

Leaver, A.G., Triffitt, J.T., Holbrook, I.B. (1975) Newer knowledge of non-collagenous protein in dentin and cortical bone matrix. *Clin. Orthop.*, **110**, 269–292.

Lippiello, L., Kaye, C., Neumata, T., Mankin, H.J. (1985) In vitro metabolic response of articular cartilage segments to low levels of hydrostatic pressure. *Connect Tissue Res.*, **13**, 99–107.

Luyten, F.P., Hascall, V.C., Nissley, S.P., Morales, T., Reddi, A.H. (1988) IGFs maintain a steady state metabolism of proteoglycans in bovine articular cartilage explants. *Arch. Biochem. Biophys.*, **267**, 416–425.

Macys, J.R., Bullough, P.G., Wilson, Jr. P.D., (1980) Coxarthrosis: a study of the natural history based on a correlation of clinical, radiographic and pathologic findings. *Semin. Arthritis Rheum.*, **10**, 66–80.

Mankin, J.H., Dorfman, H., Lippiello, L. Zarins, A. (1971) Biochemical and metabolic abnormalities in articular cartilage from osteoarthritic human hips. II. Correlation of morphology with biochemical and metabolic data. *J. Bone Joint Surg. (Am.)*, **53**: 523–537.

Maroudas, A., Evans, H., Almeida, L. (1973) Cartilage of the hip joint; topographical variation of glycosaminoglycan content in normal and fibrillated tissue. *Ann. Rheum. Dis.*, **32**, 1–9.

Matsuzawa, T., Anderson, H.C. (1971) Phosphatases of epiphyseal cartilage studied by electron microscopic cytochemical methods. *J. Histochem. Cytochem.*, **19**, 801–808.

Mayne, R., Irwin, M.H. (1986) Collagen types in cartilage. In Kuettner, K.E., Schleyerbach, R., Hascall, V.C. (Eds). *Articular cartilage biochemistry.* Raven Press, New York, 23–38.

McDevitt, C., Gilbertson, E., Muir, H. (1977) An experimental model of osteoarthritis; early morphological and biochemical changes. *J. Bone Joint Surg. (Br.)*, **59**, 24–35.

McQuillan, D.J., Handley, C.J., Campbell, M.A., Bolis, S., Milway, V.E., Herington, A.C. (1986) Stimulation of proteoglycan synthesis by IGF-1 in cultured bovine articular cartilage. *Biochem. J.*, **240**, 423–430.

Meachim, G., Collins, D.H. (1962) Cell counts of normal and osteoarthritic articular cartilage in relation to the uptake of sulphate ($^{35}SO_4$) in vitro. *Ann. Rheum. Dis.*, **21**, 45.

Moscowitz, R.W. Experimental models of osteoarthritis. In: Moskowitz, P., Howell, H., Goldberg, C., Mankin, H. (Eds) *Osteoarthritis: diagnosis and medical/surgical management*, 213–232. Saunders, Philadelphia, 1992.

Moscowitz, R.W., Goldberg, V.M. (1987) Studies of osteophyte pathogenesis in experimentally induced osteoarthritis. *J. Rheumatol.*, **14** (2), 311–320.

Muir, H., Bullough, P., Maroudas, A. (1970) The distribution of collagen in human articular cartilage with some of its physiological implications. *J. Bone Joint Surg. (Br.)*, **52**, 554–563.

Nakata, K., Bullough, P.G. (1986) The injury and repair of human articular cartilage: a morphological study of 192 cases of osteoarthritis. *Jpn. Orthop. Assoc.*, **60**: 763–775.

Ogston, A. (1876) On articular cartilage. *J. Anat. Physiol.*, **X**, 53–54.

Osbourne, K.D., Trippel, S.B., Mankin, H.J. (1989) Growth factor stimulation of adult articular cartilage. *J. Orthop. Res.*, **7**, 35–42.

Page Thomas, D.P., King, B., Stephens, T., Dingle J.T. (1991) In vivo studies of cartilage regeneration after damage induced by catabolin/ interleukin-1. *Ann. Rheum. Dis.*, **50**, 75–80.

Palmoski, M.J., Brandt, K.D. (1984) Effects of static and cyclic compressive loading on articular cartilage plugs in vitro. *Arthritis Rheum.*, **27**, 675–681.

Palmoski, M.J., Perricone, E., Brandt, K.D. (1979) Development and reversal of a proteoglycan aggregation defect in normal canine knee cartilage after immobilization. *Arthritis Rheum.*, **22**, 508–517.

Pearson, J.R., Riddell, D.M. (1962) Idiopathic osteoarthritis of the hip. *Ann. Rheum. Dis.* **21**, 31–39.

Perry, G.H., Smith, M.J.G., Whiteside, C.G. (1972) Spontaneous recovery of the joint space in degenerative hip disease. *Ann. Rheum. Dis.*, **31**, 440–448.

Rhaney, K., Lamb, D.W. (1955) The cysts of osteoarthritis of the hip. A radiological and pathological study. *J. Bone Joint Surg. (Br.)*, **37**, 663–675.

Rosenberg, L.C., Buckwalter, J.A. (1986) Cartilage proteoglycans. In Kuettner, K.E., Schleyerback, R., Hascall, V.C. (Eds). *Articular cartilage biochemistry*. Raven Press, New York, 39–57.

Sandy, J.D., Flannery, C.R., Neame, P.J., Lohmander, L.S. (1992) The structure of aggrecan fragments in human synovial fluid. *J. Clin. Invest.*, **89**, 1512–1516.

Schenk, R.K., Eggli, P.S., Hunziker, E.B. (1986) Articular cartilage morphology. In Kuettner, J., Schleyerbach R., Hascall, V. (Eds) *Articular cartilage biochemistry*. Raven Press, New York, 3–22.

Seifert, M.H., Whiteside, C.G., Savage, O. (1969) A five-year follow-up of fifty cases of idiopathic osteoarthritis of the hip. *Ann. Rheum. Dis.*, **28**, 325–326.

Stetler-Stevenson, W.G., Krutzsch, H.C., Liotta, L.A. (1989) Tissue-inhibitor of metalloproteinases (TIMP-2) a new member of the metalloproteinases inhibitor family. *J. Biol. Chem.*, **264**, 17374–17378.

Stockwell, R.A. (1979) *Biology of cartilage cells*. Cambridge University Press, Cambridge, 74.

Storey, G.O., Landells, J.W. (1971) Restoration of the femoral head after collapse in osteoarthritis. *Ann. Rheum. Dis.*, **30**, 406–412.

Tammi, M., Paukkonen, K., Kiviranta, I., Jurvelin, J., Saamanen, A.M., Helminen, H.J. (1987) Joint loading-induced alterations in articular cartilage. In *Joint loading*, Wright, Bristol, 64–88.

Termine, J.D., Belcourt, A.B., Conn, K.M., Kleinman, H.K. (1981) Mineral and collagen-binding proteins of fetal calf bone. *J. Biol. Chem.*, **256**, 10403–8.

Thonar, E.J.–M.A., Kuettner, K.E. (1987) Biochemical basis of age-related changes in proteoglycans. In Wright, T.N., Mecham, R.P. (Eds). *Biology of proteoglycans*. Academic Press, Orlando, 211–246.

Tyler, J.A., Bolis, S., Dingle, J.T., Middleton, J.F.S. (1992) Mediators of matrix metabolism. In Kuettner, K., *et al.* (Eds).*Articular cartilage and osteoarthritis*. Raven Press, New York, 251–264.

Van Der Rest, M., Garrone, R. (1991) Collagen family of proteins. FASEB J., **5**, 2814–2823.

Van Kampen, G.P.J., Vledjuijzen, J.P., Kuijer, R., Van de Stadt, R.J., Schipper, C.A. (1985) Cartilage response to mechanical force in high density chondrocyte cultures. *Arthritis Rheum.*, **28**, 419–424.

Veldhuijzen, J.P., Bourret, L.A., Rodan, G.A. (1979) In vitro studies of the effect of intermittent compressive forces on cartilage cell proliferation. *J. Cell Physiol.*, **98**: 299–306.

Villacin, A.B., Brigham, L.N., Bullough, P.G. (1979) Primary and secondary synovial chondrometaplasia. *Hum. Pathol.*, **10**: 439.

Von der Mark, K., Kirsch, T., Aigner, T., Reichenberger, E., Nerlich, A., Weseloh, G., Stob, H. (1992) The fate of chondrocytes in OA cartilage. Regeneration, de-differentiation or hypertrophy. In Kuettner, K. *et al.* (Eds). *Articular cartilage and osteoarthritis*. Raven Press, New York, 221–234.

Wilsman. N.J. (1978) Cilia of adult canine articular chondrocytes. *J. Ultrastruct. Mol. Struct. Res.*, **64**: 270–281.

Woessner, J.F. (1991) Matric metalloproteinases and their inhibitors in connective tissue remodelling. FASEB J., **5**, 2145–2154.

Wright, J.K., Cawston, T.E., Hazleman, B.L. (1991) TGFB stimulates the production of TIMP by human synovial and skin fibroblasts. *Biochim. Biophys. Acta.*, **1094**, 207–210.

Wright, J.K., Clark, I.M., Cawston, T.E., Hazleman, B.L. (1991) The secretion of TIMP by human synovial fibroblasts is modulated by all-trans-retinoic acid. *Biochem. Biophys. Acta.*, **1133**, 25–30.

4. Clinical Features and 'Subset' Characterisation

Michael Doherty

Symptoms and impact of osteoarthritis (OA)

The principal clinical manifestations of OA are:

- Symptoms – primarily pain and stiffness.
- Functional impairment.
- Signs – mainly reflecting anatomical structural change.

Although inter-related, there is often marked discordance between these three.

Symptoms

Pain is the chief complaint, though why OA should be painful is not fully understood. The absence of pain fibres in hyaline cartilage means that metabolic or structural alteration in this tissue is unlikely to be directly perceived. However, several possible mechanisms of symptom production have been suggested (**4.1**), including:

- Stimulation of pain fibres and mechanoreceptors in the capsule by intra-articular hypertension consequent upon synovial hypertrophy and increased fluid production.
- Stimulation of periosteal nerve fibres by intra-osseous hypertension (Arnoldi *et al.*, 1972).
- Perception of subchondral microfractures.
- Painful enthesopathy and bursitis that accompany structural alteration, muscle weakness and altered usage.

It has been suggested that different mechanisms may produce different pain characteristics (Hart, 1974; Kellgren, 1983). For example:

- Pain predominantly on usage – mechanical/ enthesopathy.
- Pain at rest – inflammatory.
- Pain at night – intra-osseous hypertension (a poor prognostic factor and indicator of severe damage).

However, pain may be a temporary feature of OA and can be absent in spite of severe joint damage.

Correlation between pain and radiographic change varies according to the site, being best at the hip and then the knee, with poorest correlation for hands and spinal apophyseal joints. Nevertheless, in any population, those with severe X-ray changes are more likely to have symptoms than those with mild changes – this correlation being stronger in women (Lawrence *et al.*, 1990). As with any form of pain, its subjective magnitude and perception may be greatly influenced by factors such as personality, anxiety or depression, and the business of daily activity.

Stiffness is the other chief complaint, described as 'gelling' of the joint after inactivity and difficulty in initiating movement. Prolonged morning or inactivity stiffness, often taken as a reflection of inflammation, is uncommon, but may occur particularly in patients with chronic pyrophosphate arthropathy.

Other symptoms include **joint swelling** and **deformity** (particularly of hands), and **coarse crepitus**, even in the absence of pain.

4.1

4.1 Possible sites and mechanisms of local pain production in OA.

Functional impairment

Disability results from reduced range and control of movement and from pain. Resultant handicap will vary according to individual patient requirements and aspirations. The pain and functional consequences of OA are responsible for the huge burden of morbidity in the community. Severe knee and (less commonly) hip disease both result in a massive health care problem in a generally older and otherwise fitter population.

In addition to morbidity, cumulative mortality rates among subjects aged between 55 and 74 years in the National Health and Nutrition Examination Survey (NHANES-1) were found to be significantly greater for women (but not men) with knee OA, compared to those without OA (Lawrence *et al.*, 1990). Increased mortality has also been associated with knee OA in Sweden (Danielsson and Hernborg, 1970). Although associated use of non-steroidal anti-inflammatory drugs (NSAIDs) usage may be implicated, the cause(s) remain unclear.

Signs

Crepitus (irregular articular surface), bony enlargement (osteophyte, remodelling), deformity, instability and restricted movement (with or without stress pain) may occur in any combination and primarily reflect altered joint structure (**4.2, 4.3**). Varying degrees of synovitis (warmth, effusion, synovial thickening) may accompany joint line tenderness, and muscle weakness and wasting may be apparent (**4.3–4.5**). Periarticular sources of pain, demonstrated by point tenderness away from the joint line and by stress testing, are commonly identified, particularly at the knee (inferior medial collateral ligament enthesopathy, anserine bursitis) and hip (trochanteric bursitis, gluteal enthesopathy).

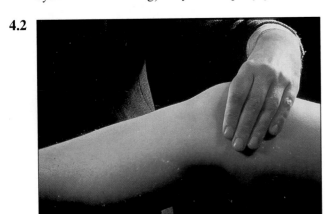

4.2 Palpable crepitus and restricted movement in OA of the knee.

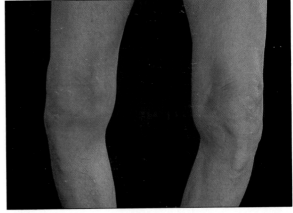

4.3 Bony enlargement (distal femora, proximal tibiae), deformity (varus), and muscle wasting (quadriceps) in bilateral knee OA.

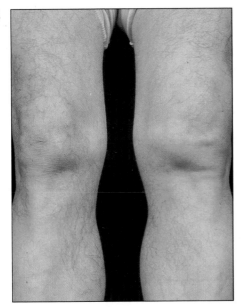

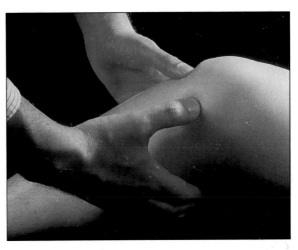

4.5 Joint line/capsular tenderness in knee OA.

4.4 Warm left knee effusion caused by accompanying synovitis in knee OA.

OA 'subsets'

The rationale for delineating groupings within 'OA', and the problems inherent in classification, are discussed in Chapter 1. Sharp distinction between these subsets does not occur. In an individual patient, evolution from one subset to another may occur with time, and at different sites. Nevertheless, such division has enabled better understanding of some of the risk factors and pathogenic mechanisms that may contribute both to the development of OA and to the tendency to 'compensate' or 'decompensate' in the face of joint insult.

Nodal generalised OA (NGOA)

This is perhaps the best recognised subset, characterised by:

- Polyarticular finger interphalangeal involvement.
- Heberden's and Bouchard's nodes.
- Female preponderance.
- Peak onset in middle age.
- Good functional outcome.
- Predisposition to OA of knee, hip, spine.
- Marked familial predisposition.

The typical patient is a woman in her 40s or 50s who develops discomfort, stiffness and swelling of a finger interphalangeal joint (IPJ). A few months later another IPJ becomes painful, then another – a 'stuttering' onset polyarthritis of distal and proximal IPJs ('monoarthritis multiplex'). Affected joints are tender and may show tight posterolateral swelling with overlying erythema (**4.6, 4.7**). Aspiration of such swellings, which initially may extend quite far proximal from the joint, may reveal viscous, clear, hyaluronate-rich 'jelly' (**4.8**): these cysts represent mucoid transformation of periarticular fibroadipose and may communicate with the joint. Typically each IPJ goes through an episodic symptom phase (over one to three years) while swelling and deformity become established; during this period hand function may be compromised. In most cases symptoms then subside, leaving the patient with typical posterolateral firm Heberden's (DIPJ) and Bouchard's (PIPJ) nodes (**4.9**), characteristic lateral subluxations of IPJs (**4.10**), and radiographic evidence of OA (**4.11**). Some patients also develop nail changes in association with florid DIPJ involvement (**4.12**).

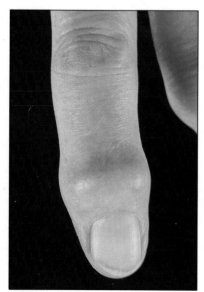

4.6 Typical posterolateral swelling of distal interphalangeal joint, with mild overlying erythema in the early stages.

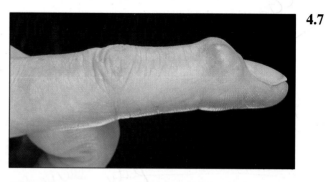

4.7 Prominent posterolateral location of Heberden's nodes.

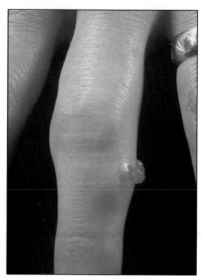

4.8 Early nodal OA, showing viscous jelly exuding from aspirated posterolateral cyst extending some distance from the joint.

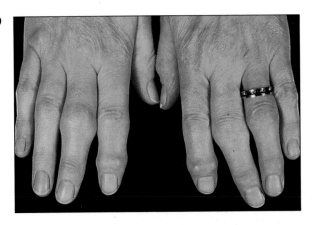

4.9 Established nodal OA showing typical Heberden's and Bouchard's nodes.

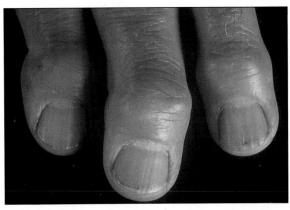

4.10 Typical lateral (radial and ulnar) deviation at distal interphalangeal joints.

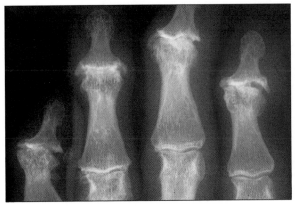

4.11 Radiographic changes (joint space loss, sclerosis, osteophyte, small osteochondral bodies or 'ossicles', lateral subluxation) in established nodal OA.

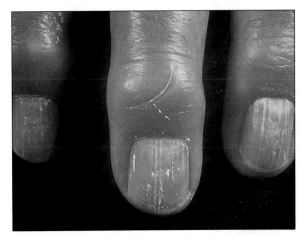

4.12 Nail dystrophy (longitudinal and transverse ridging) in fingers with distal interphalangeal nodal OA.

In addition to finger IPJs, the first carpometacarpal, metacarpophalangeal and interphalangeal joint of the thumb are commonly affected (**4.13**): other joint involvement in the hand and wrist is usually restricted to the second and third metacarpophalangeal, scaphotrapezoid (**4.14**), and pisiform-triquetral (**4.15**) articulations. The prognosis for hand OA is good; when examined two or more decades after onset, symptoms and hand function of NGOA patients are no worse than those of similarly aged subjects with no hand OA (Pattrick *et al.*, 1989a; **4.16**).

4.13

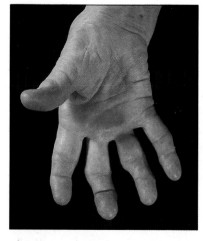

4.14

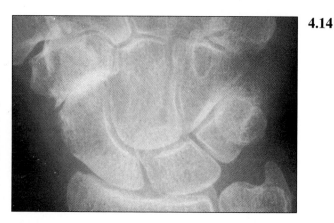

4.14 Radiograph showing OA of scaphotrapezoid joint (narrowing and sclerosis are the usual predominant changes at this site).

4.13 'Squaring' of hand (resulting from osteophyte ± subluxation) and associated global thenar muscle wasting in first carpometacarpophalangeal joint OA (note also finger interphalangeal involvement).

4.15

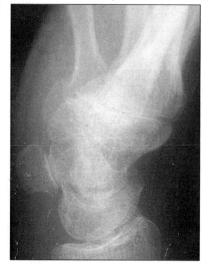

4.16

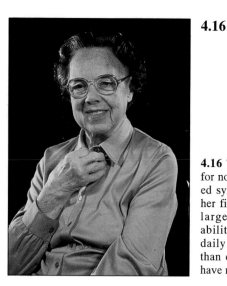

4.16 The generally good outcome for nodal OA. This patient developed symptomatic nodal hand OA in her fifties, but 20 years later she is largely asymptomatic and her ability to undertake activities of daily living is no more impaired than other women of her age who have never had hand OA.

4.15 Pisiform-triquetral OA.

Polyarticular hand IPJ OA is associated with an increased frequency of OA at other sites (Kellgren and Moore, 1952; **4.17**). This concept of 'generalised OA' was first described by Haygarth in 1805 and is supported by several studies (Roh *et al.*, 1973; Acheson and Collart, 1975; Solomon, 1983). One of these surveys (Acheson and Collart, 1975) suggests division into NGOA (nodes; DIPJ>PIPJ involvement; marked female preponderance; familial aggregation) and non-nodal generalised OA (PIPJ>DIPJ involvement; more equal sex distribution), though this distinction is not supported by others. The presence of polyarticular hand OA is associated with certain intra-articular patterns of large joint OA, for example concentric as opposed to superior pole OA of the hip (Marks, 1979), reinforcing consideration of NGOA as a separate condition. However, limited Heberden's nodes and IPJ OA are common, often asymptomatic findings in the elderly, and it may be difficult to decide when to diagnose 'NGOA'. Criteria for this subset are not widely agreed. Although 'joint involvement in at least three rays on each hand with symptoms at onset' is likely to delineate this group clearly, lesser involvement may also justify inclusion within 'NGOA'.

Although NGOA shows striking familial clustering (**4.18**), the responsible genetic factors remain unidentified. The possibility of autoimmune patho-genic mechanisms, however, is supported by the following:

- Association with HLA A1B8 (Pattrick *et al.*, 1989b).
- Female preponderance.
- Frequent onset at the menopause (hormonal modulation).
- High frequency of immune complexes in cartilage and synovium of hips (Cooke, 1985).
- High frequency of IgG rheumatoid factor positivity (but similar frequencies of Latex and Rose–Waaler positivity) and lower serum IgA levels (Hopkins *et al.*, 1992).

4.17

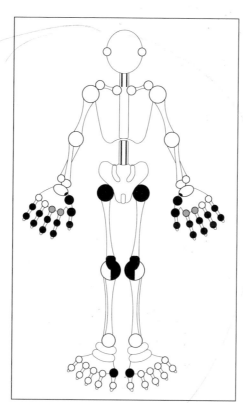

4.17 Target sites of involvement in 'generalised' nodal OA.

4.18

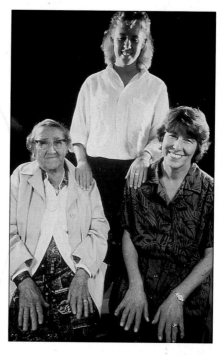

4.18 Familial predisposition in NGOA. The grandmother had self-limiting symptomatic hand OA in her fifties but continues with intermittent problems from knee OA. Her daughter is now developing symptomatic nodal OA at age 46 years, and her grand-daughter is also at increased risk of developing the same condition.

One intriguing though untested hypothesis is that a 'single-shot' (environmental?) insult in genetically and constitutionally predisposed individuals triggers an immunological response, leading to polyarticular damage and initiation of OA (**4.19**). Because it is a single temporal insult the repair process 'compensates' and results in a good outcome (Doherty *et al.*, 1990).

An alternative suggestion is that an inherited disorder of a cartilage matrix component predisposes to widespread premature joint failure. This hypothesis is supported by recent demonstration of association between alleles at the type II collagen locus COL2A1 and development of certain familial forms of generalised OA (Palotie *et al.*, 1989; Knowlton *et al.*, 1990). However, such conditions associate with or resemble epiphyseal dysplasia and show poor outcome; strong associations with COL2A1 have not been found with the more common and benign NGOA (Priestley *et al.*, 1991).

4.19

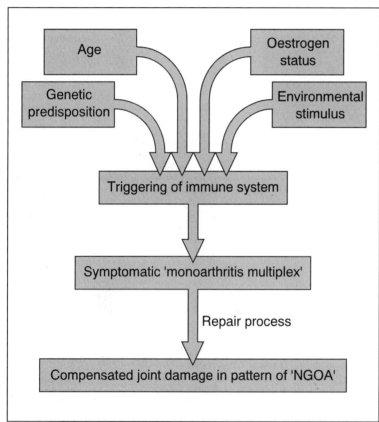

4.19 The autoimmune hypothesis for nodal OA.

Erosive ('inflammatory') OA

This rare condition is characterised by:

- Hand IPJ involvement.
- Often florid inflammatory component.
- Radiographic subchondral erosive change.
- Tendency to IPJ ankylosis.

The condition resembles NGOA in that it begins as an additive polyarthritis of finger joints (Ehlich, 1972). Inflammatory features, however, are marked and proximal and distal IPJs are equally involved. IPJ instability is common (rare in NGOA) and with occasional spontaneous IPJ ankylosis (restricted to this OA subset) the prognosis for hand function is less favourable than for nodal OA (Pattrick *et al.*, 1989a). The hallmark of this condition is the presence of subchondral erosive change (**4.20, 4.21**) which may lead to a 'gull's wing' appearance as remodelling occurs (**4.22**). Lesser degrees of erosion may prove difficult to distinguish from cysts and subchondral bony change of NGOA.

There is no predisposition to generalised OA in this subset. Microscopically the synovium is infiltrated with lymphocytes and monocytes, and pannus may be seen. The nature of this inflammatory, destructive condition is unknown, though it is of interest that similar hand changes may be associated with Sjögren's syndrome. Notably, Ehlich found that 15% of 170 patients presenting with this condition subsequently developed seropositive rheumatoid arthritis (Ehlich, 1975), bringing into question the discreteness of this subset and its place within 'OA'.

4.20

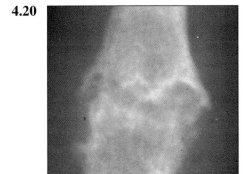

4.21

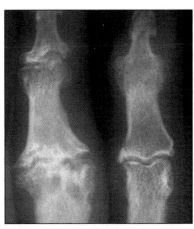

4.20 Subchondral erosive change in 'erosive OA'.

4.21 Erosive OA: subchondral erosions with loss of end plate cortical line, and DIPJ ankylosis.

4.22

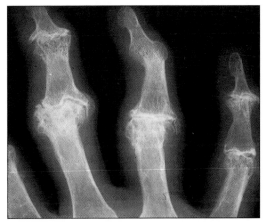

4.22 Established erosive OA, showing 'gull's wing' appearance and DIPJ ankylosis.

Large joint OA

Hip OA

Hip involvement may occur in the context of NGOA or in patients with pauciarticular large joint involvement. Subdivision is primarily on the basis of radiographic patterns, two main groups being emphasised, superior pole OA and central (medial) OA.

Superior pole OA

This common form shows focal cartilage loss in the superior part of the joint, with femoral head migration in a superolateral (most common **4.23**), superomedial (**4.24**), or directly superior (superior intermediate) direction (**4.25**). Osteophyte is most prominent at the lateral acetabular and medial femoral margins, often combined with buttressing of the medial femoral neck cortex (**4.26**). It is suggested that this pattern is:

- The more usual pattern in men.
- Mainly unilateral at presentation.
- Likely to progress (with superolateral or superomedial femoral migration). (Ledingham *et al.*, 1993.)
- Commonly secondary to local structural abnormality.

Central (medial) OA

This less common pattern shows more widespread, central cartilage loss, with less prominent femoral neck buttressing and medial or axial femoral head migration (**4.27**). It is suggested that this pattern is:

- More common in women.
- More commonly bilateral at presentation.
- The pattern that particularly associates with hand OA (Marks *et al.*, 1979).

- Less likely to progress (with axial or medial migration).

Other patterns are described (e.g. 'concentric'; **4.28**) and many patients have 'indeterminate' radiographic patterns or different patterns on the two sides. Another suggested system of classification is into 'atrophic' or 'hypertrophic' according to the balance between osteophyte and bone attrition (Solomon, 1976; Solomon, 1983; **4.29, 4.30**). Such a system is very subjective, however, and many patients are 'indeterminate' rather than clearly atrophic or hypertrophic (Ledingham *et al.*, 1993).

Suggested risk factors for hip OA include previous hip disease (e.g. Perthes' disease, slipped femoral epiphysis), acetabular dysplasia, avascular necrosis of the femoral head, severe trauma, and generalised OA. The natural history of symptomatic hip OA is poorly documented (Ledingham *et al.*, 1993). However, the general view of inevitable progression in most patients may be unwarranted. In a 10-year follow-up study Danielsson (1964) found symptom deterioration in only 17% of hip OA subjects, symptoms improving in 59%, and completely resolving in 12%; radiographic changes similarly progressed in only a minority of cases, principally those with superolateral change. Possible risk factors for progression include: superior pole pattern (Danielsson, 1964); obesity (Watson, 1976); presence of chondrocalcinosis at other sites (Menkes *et al.*, 1985); and NSAID usage (Ronningen and Langeland, 1979). Evidence for the latter, however, is far from convincing (Doherty, 1989).

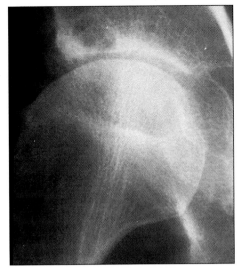

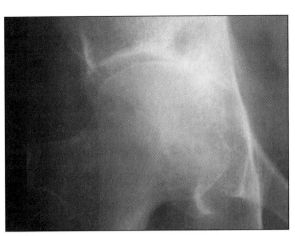

4.24 Superomedial hip OA.

4.23 Early superolateral hip OA (showing cartilage loss, acetabular cyst formation, sclerosis, mild osteophyte).

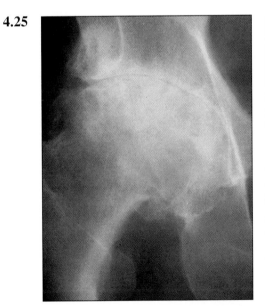

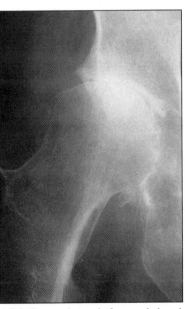

4.25 Intermediate superior pole hip OA: changes are widespread and advanced but predominantly associated with superior femoral head migration.

4.26 Superolateral femoral head migration with typical 'buttressing' of medial femoral neck (periosteal osteophyte).

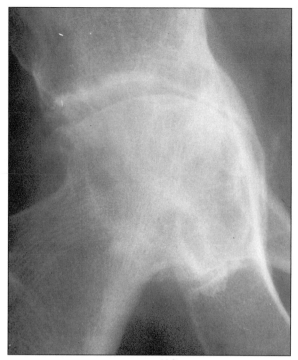

4.28 'Concentric' hip OA (a rare pattern).

4.27 Medial pattern of hip OA.

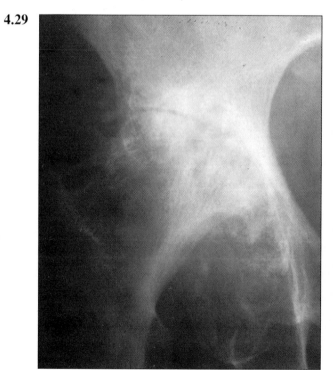

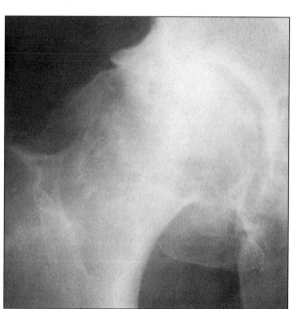

4.30 Hypertrophic hip OA – osteophyte and bone remodelling are the predominant changes.

4.29 Atrophic hip OA – the balance of change being towards marked bone and cartilage attrition.

Knee OA

The knee is a commonly affected site. Involvement is often bilateral, particularly in women and in the elderly, and shows strong association with hand OA (Kellgren and Moore, 1952; Acheson and Collart, 1975; Cushnaghan and Dieppe, 1991). Population surveys show most frequent involvement of the medial tibiofemoral compartment (**4.31**), with varus the most characteristic deformity (**4.32**). The patellofemoral compartment, however, is often omitted from large studies, but when included appears equally if not more commonly involved (both symptomatically and radiographically; **4.33**).

Risk factors for development of knee OA include:

- Previous trauma/mechanical insult (e.g. meniscectomy).
- Obesity (Felson, 1988).
- Generalised OA.
- Distal femoral dysplasia (Cooke, 1985).
- Female gender.

Smoking may be protective at this site (Felson, 1988; Samanta *et al.*, 1993). The natural history of knee OA may be less favourable than that for hips. Hernborg and Nilsson (1977) observed clinical and radiographic deterioration in most cases followed for 10 to 18 years; varus deformity, earlier age of onset, and female gender were related to worse prognosis. Isolated osteophyte alone was shown not to be associated with subsequent development of OA. In addition to increased morbidity, knee OA is associated with increased mortality (Danielsson and Hernborg, 1970; Lawrence *et al.*, 1990).

4.31

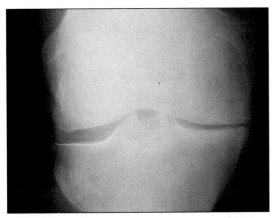

4.31 Knee OA, predominating in the medial tibiofemoral compartment.

4.32

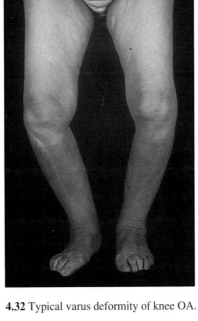

4.32 Typical varus deformity of knee OA.

4.33

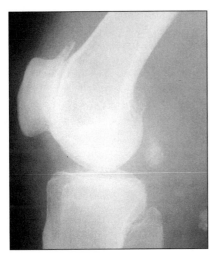

4.33 Patellofemoral OA—a common finding, and a common source of knee symptoms.

Crystal-associated subsets

A number of particles are commonly identified in OA joints, most notably calcium pyrophosphate dihydrate (CPPD) and apatite (carbonated hydroxyapatite and other basic calcium phosphates). The origin and role of such particles in the OA process remain unknown (Doherty and Dieppe, 1988; Dieppe *et al.*, 1988). It was initially assumed that such crystals were injurious and the cause of specific 'crystal deposition disease' (McCarty, 1976). Certainly CPPD and apatite are demonstrably inflammatory agents, and being particulate could exert deleterious mechanical effects. However, the common occurrence of calcium crystals in asymptomatic, otherwise normal joints, and lack of disease specificity, have questioned such a role. In the context of OA, it seems more likely that CPPD and apatite reflect underlying metabolic or physical facets of the OA process, potentially acting as markers for differing forms of joint response.

Pyrophosphate arthropathy

CPPD crystal deposition is the commonest cause of chondrocalcinosis (**4.34**). Although familial and metabolic disease predisposition are recognised, CPPD deposition most commonly occurs as an apparently sporadic, age-related phenomenon. Although commonly an asymptomatic, incidental finding (Doherty and Dieppe, 1988), the two common clinical presentations are chronic arthropathy and acute synovitis.

Chronic pyrophosphate arthropathy

This common subset is characterised by:

- Predominance in elderly females.
- Often florid inflammatory component (± super-imposed acute attacks).
- The knee as the target joint.
- Frequent involvement of joints and joint compartments uncommonly affected by OA.
- Frequent 'hypertrophic' radiographic appearance.
- Calcification of articular structures.
- Synovial fluid CPPD crystals (**4.35**).

The knees are the most commonly and severely affected site, followed by wrists, shoulders, elbows, hips, mid-tarsal and ankle joints (**4.36**). Metacarpophalangeal joints (particularly second and third) are a commonly affected site in the hand (**4.37**). Symptoms are usually confined to a few joints, though single or multiple joint involvement also occurs; acute attacks may be superimposed upon chronic symptoms. Affected joints show signs of OA (bony swelling, crepitus, restricted movement) with varying degrees of inflammation. Synovitis may be marked, particularly at the knee (**4.38**), radiocarpal and glenohumeral joints. Knees typically show involvement of two or three compartments, with marked, usually predominant patellofemoral disease. In severe cases fixed flexion with either valgus or varus deformity may occur (**4.39**).

Radiographic changes of arthropathy are those of OA, but characteristics which may permit distinction include:

- Joint distribution (wrist, shoulder, elbow, ankle) and involvement within articulations (e.g. predominant patellofemoral disease) atypical of uncomplicated OA.
- Prominent, exuberant osteophyte and cyst formation.

These may present a distinctive 'hypertrophic' appearance and distribution that suggest CPPD even in the absence of chondrocalcinosis (**4.40**). Chondrocalcinosis most commonly affects fibrocartilage (particularly knee menisci, wrist triangular cartilage, symphysis pubis), but also occurs in hyaline cartilage as thick linear deposits parallel to and separate from subchondral bone (**4.41**); it may be localised, but usually affects several joints. Calcification of capsule, synovium and tendon is less common (**4.42**, **4.43**).

Acute synovitis ('pseudogout')

The typical attack develops rapidly with severe pain and swelling, maximal within 6 to 24 hours of onset. Examination reveals a tender joint, signs of marked synovitis, and often overlying erythema (**4.44**). Fever is common, and elderly patients may be unwell and confused. Diagnosis rests on the finding of synovial fluid CPPD crystals and exclusion of sepsis. Attacks are self-limiting, usually resolving within one to three weeks. Although most episodes develop spontaneously, several provoking factors are recognised:

- Intercurrent illness (e.g. chest infection).
- Direct trauma to joint.
- Surgery (especially parathyroidectomy).
- Blood transfusion, parenteral fluid administration.
- Institution of thyroxine replacement therapy.
- Joint lavage.

The natural history of pyrophosphate arthropathy is poorly documented. However, one 5-year prospective study found that most patients run a benign course (Doherty *et al.*, 1993). Even in severely affected knees (the usual presenting site), 60% showed stabilisation or improvement of symptoms; similarly, the commonest radiographic change was an increase in osteophytes with bone remodelling. Nevertheless, severe progressive 'destructive pyrophosphate arthropathy' of large joints occasionally occurs; this is virtually confined to elderly women and may be associated with problematic recurrent haemarthrosis (**4.45**).

A number of associations with CPPD crystal deposition are recognised (**Table 4.1**). Several observations support a relationship between preceding joint insult and subsequent CPPD deposition; for example, the high frequency of chondrocalcinosis in post-meniscectomy knees (Doherty *et al.*, 1982). The negative association between CPPD and rheumatoid,

Table 4.1 Associations of CPPD crystal deposition.

Positive	
	Ageing
	Familial predisposition
	Metabolic disease
	Joint insult, OA
	(DISH)
Negative	
	Rheumatoid arthritis

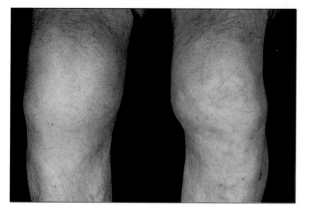

4.44 Acute pseudogout of the knee, showing marked synovitis with tense effusion and overlying erythema.

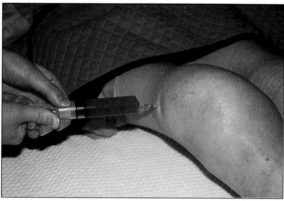

4.45 Blood-stained synovial fluid is a common finding in chronic pyrophosphate arthropathy during episodes of pseudogout or when associated with destructive change.

however, with atypical radiographic features in patients with coexistent disease, suggest the primary association is with hypertrophic tissue response/OA rather than joint damage per se. This might in part explain the exuberant osteophytosis and remodelling, and generally good outcome in pyrophosphate arthropathy. Factors accompanying hypertrophic OA that predispose to CPPD are unknown, though alterations in pyrophosphate levels and in matrix factors (inhibitors or promotors of crystal nucleation and growth) may both be involved. For example, synovial fluid pyrophosphate levels are elevated in OA but reduced in rheumatoid, perhaps reflecting increased chondrocyte activity and division in OA. Equally, possible promoting roles for collagen and acidic phospholipid, with reduction in inhibitory proteoglycan, may be relevant.

Apatite-associated arthropathy

This uncommon condition is characterised by:

- Confinement to elderly, predominantly female subjects.
- Localisation to large joints (**4.46**).
- Rapid progression of arthropathy with instability.
- Marked attrition of cartilage and bone.
- Abundant apatite in synovial fluid and synovium.

This condition has a number of synonyms, including 'Milwaukee shoulder' and 'basic calcium phosphate deposition disease' (Halverson and McCarty, 1988). Typical patients are elderly women with rapidly progressive arthropathy of the hip, shoulder or knee; usually only one or a few sites are affected. Onset is often sudden. Within a few weeks or months the patient has severe rest and night pain, and shows large, cool effusions with gross instability (**4.47**). Aspirated synovial fluid is often blood-stained and shows retained viscosity and modest increase in cells; alizarin red S staining at acidic pH shows multiple calcium-containing aggregates (**4.48**), confirmed as apatite by more definitive means. The main radiographic features are marked attrition of cartilage and bone, with paucity of osteophyte and sclerosis – a markedly 'atrophic' appearance (**4.49**). The differential diagnosis includes late avascular necrosis, sepsis and atrophic Charcot arthropathy. The prognosis is poor, most patients coming to arthroplasty.

The pathogenesis of this arthropathy is a matter of controversy (Halverson and McCarty, 1988). McCarty and colleagues have emphasised the presence of activated collagenase in synovial fluid, a proliferative response to crystals by synoviocytes, and the frequency of accompanying periarticular calcification, suggesting that apatite deposited in capsule and periarticular structures is enzymatically 'strip-mined'. The free apatite then interacts with synoviocytes, resulting in further collagenase release, further strip-mining and progression of arthropathy and instability via an 'amplification loop' mechanism (**4.50**). Others, however, have not confirmed an increase in collagenase activities, and suggest that the apatite primarily originates from subchondral and marginal bone (Doherty and Dieppe, 1988). The nonspecific finding of apatite in other arthropathies (and even in small amounts in normal joints) is consistent with this interpretation, the amount of apatite simply reflecting the rapidity of bone damage. Other hypotheses, for example that it results from NSAID usage and is a specific 'iatrogenic Charcot arthropathy', seem less plausible (Doherty, 1989).

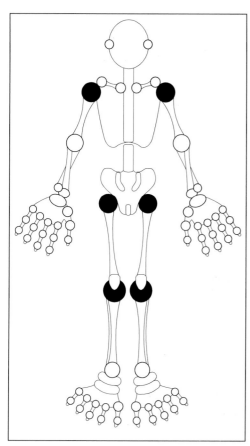

4.46 Target sites for apatite-associated destructive arthritis.

4.47 Apatite-associated destructive arthropathy affecting the shoulder of an 80-year-old woman who has had symptoms for eight months. Note the large, cool effusion evident in the subacromial/subdeltoid bursa.

4.48 Alizarin red positive particles in synovial fluid from the patient in **4.47**.

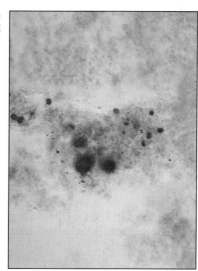

4.49 Apatite-associated destructive arthritis of hip. This radiograph was taken four months after onset of hip symptoms and shows marked attrition both sides of the joint, apparent widening of joint space, and paucity of osteophyte.

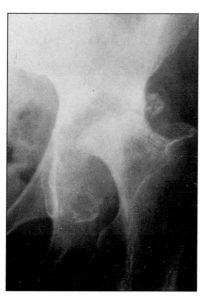

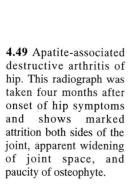

4.50 One hypothesis to explain apatite-associated destructive arthritis (McCarty *et al.*).

79

e frequent occurrence of these calcium crystals in the me joint (concurrent or during differing phases) or in ifferent joints of the same individual is not nexpected. In joints showing a preponderance of ither hypertrophic or atrophic change (i.e. the two nds of the OA spectrum) the likelihood of a single crystal species would be higher (**4.51**).

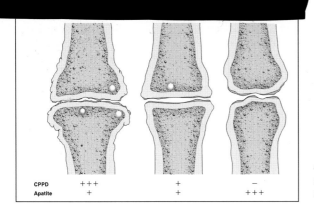

CPPD	+++	+	−
Apatite	+	+	+++

4.51 The spectrum of crystal deposition in OA, with CPPD associating with 'hypertrophic', generally good outcome OA, and apatite with 'atrophic', bad outcome OA.

OA at other joint sites

Selection of OA for certain joint sites is striking. For example, compared to OA of interphalangeal joints, hips or knees, OA of the elbow, glenohumeral joint or ankle is unusual and principally confined to older subjects. As with other arthropathies, the distribution of OA remains largely unexplained.

OA of spinal apophyseal joints (particularly lower cervical and lower lumbar segments), first carpometacarpal and first metatarsophalangeal joints is common (**4.52**), occurring as part of generalised OA or as an isolated feature. NGOA and trauma are predisposing factors at all three sites. Additional associations include:

• Metatarsus primus varus (first MTPJ).

• Congenital structural anomalies, adjacent spondylosis deformans, and hip OA (apophyseal joints).

Elbow OA may occur in patients with NGOA and pyrophosphate arthropathy, but in the absence of these it is usually explained in terms of repetitive, principally occupational, trauma. The same applies to OA of second and third metacarpophalangeal joints ('Missouri arthropathy'). Recent surveys, however, suggest that elbow and metacarpophalangeal joint OA may occur particularly in men (**4.53, 4.54**), be associated with a good prognosis, and be largely unrelated to trauma or handedness (Doherty and Preston, 1989; Cushnaghan and Dieppe, 1991).

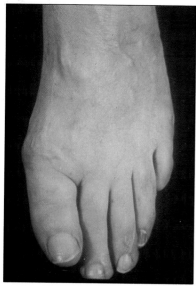

4.52 First MTPJ osteoarthritis with associated mild hallux valgus and rotation deformity, and overlying bunion.

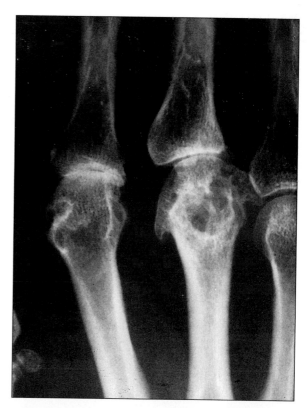

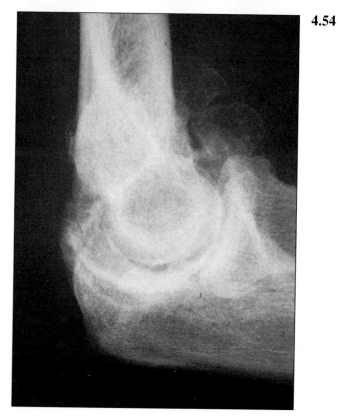

4.53, 4.54 Association of elbow and MCPJ osteoarthritis.

OA as part of other disease

Because OA may represent the repair process of synovial joints, it is expected that features of OA will be involved during certain phases of other defined arthropathies. A common example is rheumatoid arthritis, when limited osteophytosis, sclerosis and remodelling may 'superimpose' during later, less inflammatory periods of the disease (**4.55, 4.56**). In such instances 'OA' is better, and more generally, accepted as an accompanying process of tissue response/repair rather than an acquired second condition.

The same applies to other inflammatory, metabolic or structural arthropathies that damage joints and trigger repair (*see* Chapter 10). Ochronosis and spondylo-epiphyseal dysplasia are sometimes included within the umbrella of OA, but are in fact examples of successful recognition of triggering factors (diseases) that allow removal from the 'OA' classification; endemic forms of OA similarly merit consideration in their own right. For clinical purposes, however, it is still useful to consider together conditions that may result in non-inflammatory arthropathy with radiographic changes predominantly of OA. Despite some overlap, these are probably best grouped by clinical presentation (**Table 4.2**). Clinical features of arthropathy that should suggest consideration of predisposing disease include:

- Premature onset OA (younger than 45 years).
- Atypical joint distribution (e.g. prominent metacarpophalangeal and radiocarpal involvement in haemochromatosis).
- Premature onset chondrocalcinosis (younger than 55 years).
- Florid polyarticular chondrocalcinosis (any age).

Such patients usually have other clinical or radiographic clues, and routine 'screening' of patients with OA or chondrocalcinosis for all known predisposing diseases (many of which are rare) is inappropriate.

Table 4.2 Principal conditions with presentations and radiographic changes that may stimulate OA

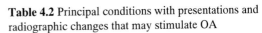

1 Generalised 'OA'
   (Spondylo-) epiphyseal dysplasia
   Ochronosis
   Haemochromatosis
   Wilson's disease
   Endemic OA (e.g. Kashin Beck disease)

2 Pauciarticular, large joint 'OA'
   Acromegaly
   Neuropathic joints:
      Syringomyelia – shoulders, wrists, elbows
      Diabetes – hindfoot, midfoot
      Tabes – knees, spine
   Avascular necrosis (mainly proximal and distal femur, proximal humerus)

4.55

4.56

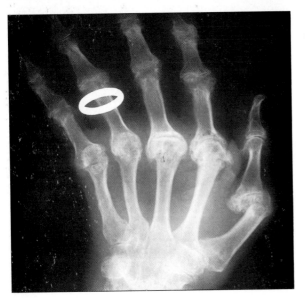

4.55 The left hand of a 74-year-old woman with rheumatoid arthritis for 40 years. Her hand symptoms had been stable for eight years. Bony swelling and painless restriction of movement, with little evidence of synovitis, were the main examination findings.

4.56 Hand radiograph of the patient in **4.55** showing osteophyte and bone remodelling ('repair') superimposed upon erosive damage caused by rheumatoid arthritis.

References and further reading

Acheson, R.M., Collart, A.B. (1975) New Haven survey of joint diseases. XVII. Relationships between some systemic characteristics and osteoarthrosis in a general population. *Ann. Rheum. Dis.*, **34**, 379–387.

Arnoldi, C.C., Linderholm, H., Mussbicheler, H. (1972) Venous engorgement and intraosseous hypertension in osteoarthritis of the hip. *J. Bone Joint Surg.*, **54B**, 409–421.

Cooke, T.D.V. (1985) Pathogenic mechanisms in poly-articular osteoarthritis. *Clin. Rheum. Dis.*, **11**(2), 203–238.

Cushnaghan, J., Dieppe, P. (1991) Study of 500 patients with limb joint osteoarthritis. I. Analysis by age, sex, and distribution of symptomatic joint sites. *Ann. Rheum. Dis.*, **50**, 8–13.

Danielsson, L.G. (1964) Incidence and prognosis of coxarthrosis. *Acta Orthop. Scand.*, Suppl. 66, 1–114.

Danielsson, L.G., Hernborg, J. (1970) Morbidity and mortality of osteoarthritis of the knee (gonarthrosis) in Malmo, Sweden. *Clin. Orthop. Rel. Res.*, **69**, 224–226.

Dieppe, P.A., Campion, G., Doherty, M. (1988) Mixed crystal deposition. *Rheum. Dis. Clin. N. Am.*, **14**, 415–426.

Doherty, M. (1989) Chondroprotection by NSAIDs. *Ann. Rheum. Dis.*, **48**, 619–621.

Doherty, M., Dieppe, P.A. (1988) Clinical aspects of calcium pyrophosphate dihydrate crystal deposition. *Rheum. Dis. Clin. N. Am.*, **14**, 395–414.

Doherty, M., Preston, B. (1989) Primary osteoarthritis of the elbow. *Ann. Rheum. Dis.*, **48**, 743–747.

Doherty, M., Watt, I., Dieppe, P.A. (1982) Localised chondrocalcinosis in post-meniscectomy knees. *Lancet*, **i**, 1207–1210.

Doherty, M., Pattrick, M., Powell, R.J. (1990) Hypothesis – nodal generalised osteoarthritis is an auto-immune disease. *Ann. Rheum. Dis.*, **49**, 1017–1020.

Doherty, M., Dieppe, P.A., Watt, I. (1993) Pyrophosphate arthropathy: a prospective study. *Br. J. Rheumatol.*, **32**, 189–196.

Ehlich, G.E. (1972) Inflammatory osteoarthritis: I. The clinical syndrome. *J. Chron. Dis.*, **25**, 317–328.

Ehlich, G.E. (1975) Osteoarthritis beginning with inflammation, definitions and correlations. *JAMA*, **232**, 157–159.

Felson, D.T. (1988) Epidemiology of hip and knee osteoarthritis. *Epidem. Rev.*, **10**, 1–28.

Halverson, P.B., McCarty, D.J. (1988) Clinical aspects of basic calcium phosphate crystal deposition. *Rheum. Dis. Clin. N. Am.*, **14**(2), 427–439.

Hart, F.D. (1974) Pain in osteoarthritis. *Practitioner*, **212**, 244–250.

Hernborg, J.S., Nilsson, B.E. (1977) The natural course of untreated osteoarthritis of the knee. *Clin. Orthop. Rel. Res.*, **123**, 130–137.

Hopkinson, N., Powell, R.J., Doherty, M. (1992) Auto-antibodies, immunoglobulins and Gm allotypes in nodal generalised osteoarthritis. *Br. J. Rheumatol.*, **31**, 605–608.

Kellgren, J.H. (1983) Pain in osteoarthritis. *J. Rheumatol.*, **10** (suppl. 9), 108–109.

Kellgren, J.H., Moore, R. (1952) Generalised osteoarthritis and Heberden's nodes. *Br. Med. J.*, **1**, 181–187.

Knowlton, R.G., Katzenstein, P.L., Moskovitz, R.W., Malemud, C.J., Pathria, M.N., Jimenez, S.A., Prockop, D.J. (1990) Genetic linkage of a polymorphism in the type II procollagen gene (COL2A1) to primary osteoarthritis associated with mild chondrodysplasia. *N. Engl. J. Med.*, **22**, 526–530.

Lawrence, R.C., Everett, D., Hochberg, M.C. (1990) Arthritis. In *Health Status and Well-being of the Elderly: National Health and Nutrition Examination – Epidemiologic Follow-up Survey.* Huntley, R., Cornoni-Huntley, J. (eds.), 136–151, Oxford University Press, New York.

Ledingham, J., Dawson, S., Preston, B., Doherty, M. (1993) Radiographic progression of hospital referred osteoarthritis of the hip. *Ann. Rheum. Dis.*, **52**, 263–267.

Marks, J.S., Stewart, I.M., Hardinge, K. (1979) Primary osteoarthrosis of the hip and Heberden's nodes. *Ann. Rheum. Dis.*, **38**, 107–111.

McCarty, D.J. (1976) Calcium pyrophosphate dihydrate crystal deposition disease – 1975. *Arthritis Rheum.*, **19** (suppl.), 275–286.

Menkes, C-J., Decraemere W., Postel, M., Forest, M. (1985) Chondrocalcinosis and rapid destruction of the hip. *J. Rheumatol.*, **12**, 130–133.

Palotie, A., Vaisanen, P., Ott, J., Ryhanen, L., Elima, K., Vikkula, M., Cheah, K., Vuorio, E., Peltonen, L. (1989) *Lancet*, **i**, 924–927.

Pattrick, M., Aldridge, S., Hamilton, E., Manhire, A., Doherty, M. (1989a) A controlled study of hand function in nodal and erosive osteoarthritis. *Ann. Rheum. Dis.*, **48**, 978–982.

Pattrick, M., Manhire, A., Milford-Ward, A., Doherty, M. (1989b) HLA AB antigens and alpha-1-antitrypsin phenotypes in nodal generalised osteoarthritis and erosive osteoarthritis. *Ann. Rheum. Dis.*, **48**, 470–475.

Priestley, L., Fergusson, C., Ogilvie, D., Wordsworth, P., Smith, R., Pattrick, M., Doherty, M., Sykes, B. (1991) A limited association of generalised OA with alleles at the type II collagen locus: COL2A1. *Br. J. Rheumatol.*, **30**, 272–275.

Roh, Y.S., Dequecker, J., Mulier, J.C. (1973) Osteoarthrosis at the hand skeleton in primary osteoarthrosis of the hip and in normal controls. *Clin. Orthop.*, **90**, 90–94.

Ronningen, H., Langeland, N. (1979) Indomethacin treatment in osteoarthritis of the hip joint. Does the treatment interfere with the natural course of the disease? *Acta Orthop. Scand.*, **50**, 169–174.

Solomon, L. (1976) Patterns of osteoarthritis of the hip. *J. Bone Joint Surg.*, **58B**, 176–183.

Solomon, L. (1983) Osteoarthritis, local and generalised: a uniform disease? *J. Rheumatol.*, **10** (suppl. 9), 13–15.

Watson, M. (1976) Femoral head height loss: a study of the relative significance of some of its determinants in hip degeneration. *Rheumatol. Rehabil.*, **15**, 264–269.

5. Radiology and Imaging

Iain Watt

"He who first gave names, gave them according to his conception of the things which they signified, and if his conception was erroneous shall we not be deceived by him?"

Osteoarthritis (OA) is frequently diagnosed, classified and staged on the basis of X-ray examinations. The features used to substantiate that diagnosis are classical and include eburnation, osteophytosis, narrowing of the distance between the bone ends ('joint space narrowing'), joint effusion, capsular thickening and deformity (**5.1**). These features, indeed their very names, are derived from morbid pathology (**5.2**). This practice is dangerous, however, because on a radiograph one does not see eburnation, but increased subcortical bone density; not 'cysts' but radiolucencies which *may* be cysts; and the space between bone ends *could* represent cartilage thickness, but may not. There is also serious disparity between the features of OA assessed visually and bones recovered from archaeological sites and the radiographic assessment thereof (Rogers *et al.*, 1990).

The whole spectrum of radiological technologies can be applied to the study of OA. For convenience, however, these may be divided into those that demonstrate apparent anatomy (this includes plain films and various modifications thereof) and those that demonstrate the current physiological status of the joint (including radionuclide and magnetic resonance imaging [MRI]). This distinction is of considerable importance because a plain film provides a static anatomical record of events which occurred weeks or months previously. Hence when a patient presents with an acutely painful joint and radiographic features which have not shown any recent change, one should not be lulled into a sense of false security. Rapid change may be occurring in that joint, which the more physiological investigations can reveal (Cobby *et al.*, 1989).

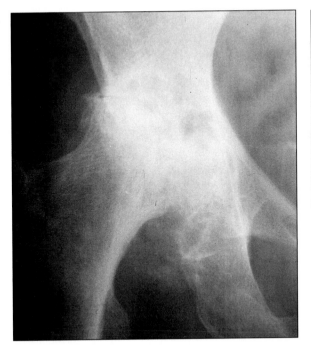

5.1 Typical OA of the hip joint. Superolateral migration is demonstrated with extensive osteophytosis, subchondral sclerosis, bone attrition, subchondral sclerosis, bone attrition, subchondral radiolucencies and obvious deformity.

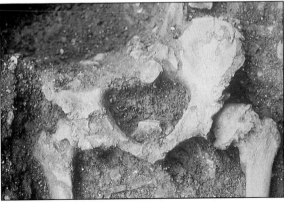

5.2 At this archaeological excavation, typical OA at the left hip is demonstrated. Note the hypertrophic osteophytosis and the obvious adduction and flexion deformity. (Courtesy of Dr Juliet Rogers.)

In this chapter the author seeks to challenge the concept that OA is simply a progressive, degenerative 'wear and tear' phenomenon, as well as pointing to the inadequacies of using a pathology model to interpret radiographs. Osteoarthritis is not a uniform disease nor is it possible to predict the manifestations of OA within an individual joint. Accordingly, classifications of disease status, such as those of Kellgren and Lawrence (1957), are woefully inadequate, for the following reasons:

- The classical features of joint space narrowing, juxta-articular osteophytes, intra-articular loose bodies and joint swelling are age-related phenomena (Makela *et al.*, 1979). Ageing is associated with cartilage thinning and reduced bone mass. Furthermore, increased congruity of the joints occurs alongside a reduction in function. Consequently, joint space narrowing may be regarded as an age-related phenomenon, and the osteophytosis developed from chondrophyte on the margins of joints in order to improve stability. Neither of these indicate 'disease' (**5.3**). It has been suggested (**5.4**) that the increased congruity of the joint reduces hyaline cartilage nutrition, which promotes degenerative change and subsequent bony abnormality.

- Even allowing for the age-related phenomena, there is a far from uniform radiological appearance in individual joints (**5.5–5.7**). Whilst all the classical signs may be present in a joint (**5.5**), only osteophyte (**5.6**) or joint space narrowing (**5.7**) may predominate.

- Even were hyaline cartilage thinning deemed to be the single most important feature of OA, it is very difficult to assess on plain film because the radiograph demonstrates articular cortices. The gap between, in theory, could contain anything, from joint fluid to synovium and cartilage.

5.3

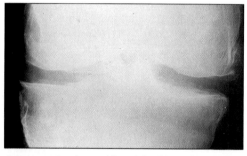

5.3 Age-related osteophyte? In this patient, a film taken weight-bearing, minor rim osteophytosis is demonstrated in both compartments. Note the slightly rounded tibial spines but preserved joint space width. Is this disease or normal ageing?

5.

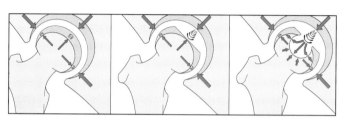

5.4 The concept of increasing congruity, change in loading and cartilage nutrition is illustrated. Hyaline cartilage at the apex of the spherical joint head is thinned with subsequent damage to underlying bone (after P. Bullough).

5.6

5.5

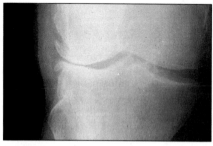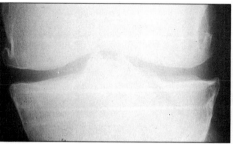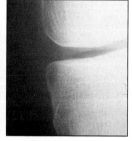

5.

5.5–5.7 The spectrum of change in OA of the knee is demonstrated. **5.5** Hypertrophic, lateral compartment OA with obvious joint space narrowing, abundant rim osteophytosis and subarticular sclerosis. **5.6** Here joint space width is preserved with no evidence of abnormal subchondral sclerosis. However, there is abundant rim osteophytosis. **5.7** A chance 'vacuum' sign demonstrates obvious hyaline cartilage thinning in this medial compartment. However there are no other features of OA.

Methods of coping with these problems include:

- **Weight-bearing films**. By imaging under conditions of load (weight bearing) it may be assumed that articular surfaces will be in contact and hence the interbone gap represents cartilage thickness. Whilst this has no great value in the hip, it is extremely helpful in the knee. A load line exists between the femoral heads, tibial spines and tali as originally illustrated by Leonardo da Vinci (**5.8**)! Radiographically, this may also be recorded using three hinged films in a long cassette (**5.9**). Decreased joint space, 2mm or more, will be expected in one or either compartment assessed by this means in preoperative patients with osteoarthritis (Leach *et al.*, 1970).
- Even with weight bearing, a true sense of joint space narrowing may not be achieved and subsequently, **stress films** may be used (Gibson and Goodfellow, 1986) (**5.10**, **5.11**). Occasionally quite dramatic results can be obtained (**5.12**).
- Hyaline cartilage thickness can be demonstrated accurately by introducing **contrast medium** into the relevant joint (Hall and Wyshack, 1980), normative data in the knee having been established. Hyaline cartilage width can be demonstrated accurately (**Table 5.1**, **5.13**) and focal defects demonstrated (**5.14**).
- It is often not practicable to introduce contrast medium in a joint. **Adaptations of radiographic technique** may help to assess joint space narrowing more accurately: for example, a degree of knee flexion is desirable (Rosenberg *et al.*, 1988) (**5.15**).

In all of these methods magnification will account for between 25 and 40% of any error in measurement (Hall and Wyshack, 1980).

5.8

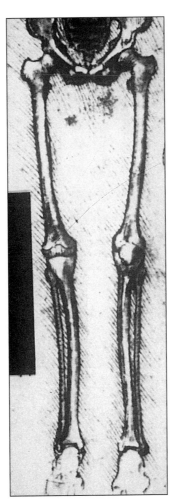

5.9

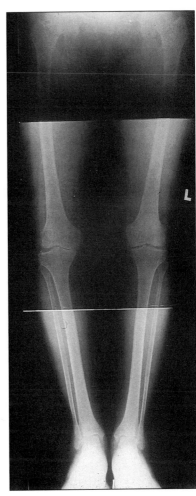

5.8 The normal load line is demonstrated from an original drawing by Leonardo da Vinci. Notice that the femoral heads, tibial spines and ankle mortise form a straight line.

5.9 A clinical load line radiograph is demonstrated. Three hinged films are placed in a cassette and, in order to cope with differing thickness of body and therefore exposure factors, graded screens are used in the cassettes. Overall an excellent demonstration of load line and deformity can be obtained. Note modest medial compartment OA on the right.

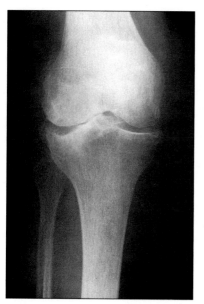
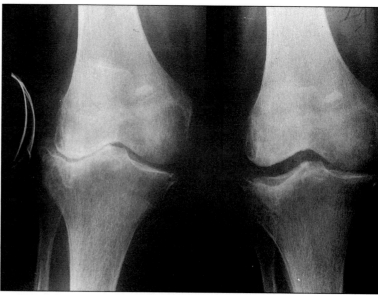

5.10, 5.11 Stress films. **5.10** A conventional weight-bearing film, whilst demonstrating some features of OA in the lateral compartment, suggests that joint space width is not particularly narrowed. **5.11** Varus and valgus stress films demonstrate the truth to be quite different, however. Valgus stress shows that the lateral compartment is almost completely narrowed and that there is some distraction of the lateral compartment on varus stressing. Hence, even in the weight-bearing position, this patient seemed to be balancing on the tibial spines.

5.12

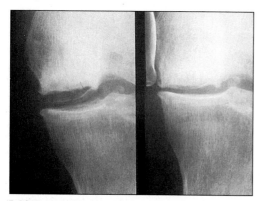

Table 5.1 Normative data for hyaline cartilage thickness as measured (in mm) at knee arthrography (after Hall and Wyshack, 1980).

	Medial	Lateral	Ages (years)
Male	4.3 ± .7	3.9 ± 13.7	33.9 ± 13.7
Female	3.6 ± .7	3.3 ± .7	36.1 ± 15.8

5.12 Stress films in avascular necrosis. Here a patient with idiopathic medial femoral condyle necrosis was undergoing assessment preoperatively. In varus stressing, joint space narrowing is shown to be considerable. However, in valgus stressing the femoral condylar cartilage and an underlying sliver of cortical bone are shown to be loosened and separate within the zone of avascular necrosis.

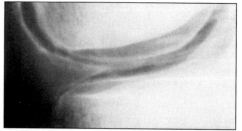

5.13

5.13 Normal medial compartment knee arthrography demonstrates clearly hyaline cartilage thickness and outlines the anterior horn of the medial meniscus.

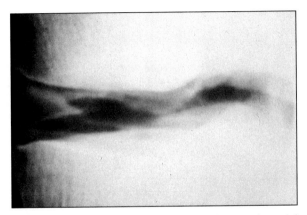

5.14

5.14 Medial compartment knee arthrography. A substantial hyaline cartilage defect is demonstrated on the femoral condyle. This was clinically unsuspected in a patient with medial compartment knee pain.

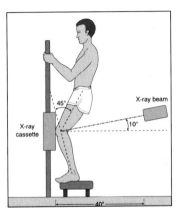

5.15

5.15 More accurate assessment of knee joint space narrowing may be obtained using a degree of knee flexion (after Rosenberg *et al.*, 1988).

Radiologically, however, OA resembles a spectrum. In the hip, for example, several major forms exist including superior polar (**5.16**, **5.17**), concentric (**5.18**) and rarer variants such as predominant subchondral cyst/geode formation (**5.19**) which, when laterally placed, presents as a mass lesion or Eggar's cyst (**5.20**, **5.21**). Whilst much attention has been paid to the role of the femoral head articular cartilage in hip OA, it is worth remembering that disease may begin radiographically in the acetabular roof (**5.22**). Furthermore, the degree and type of bone response also covers a spectrum from a very hypertrophic form (**5.23**) to that of an atrophic destructive type (**5.24**).

The challenge radiographically, therefore, is to classify and subset OA rather than to lump it together in one progressive, predictable disease state.

5.16

5.16, 5.17 Superior polar hip OA. Note the typical superolateral migration, attrition of the acetabular roof, superolateral sclerosis and attrition of bone. **5.17** This hip was not dysplastic developmentally. About 2 years previously it was essentially normal (**5.16**) save for a slight superior joint space narrowing.

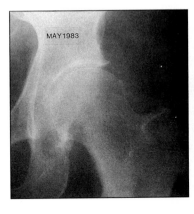

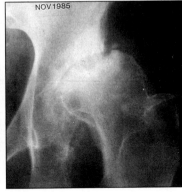

5.17

5.18

5.18 Typical bilateral concentric hip OA. Note the deep moulded acetabuli, the minor degree of protrusion, the 'jet stream' type osteophytes and yet relatively preserved joint space width.

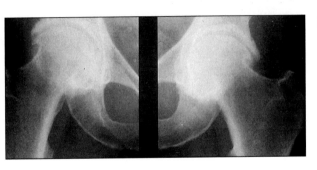

5.19

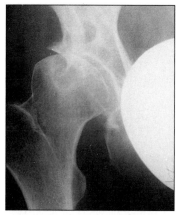

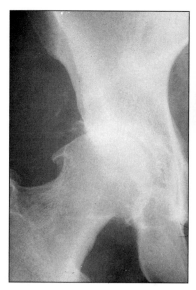

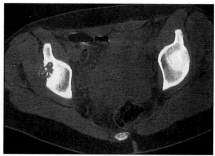

5.20, 5.21 Eggar's cyst. **5.20** Demonstrates concentric hip OA with erosive ill-defined ossification in the soft tissues adjacent to the acetabular roof. **5.21** CT confirms the presence of an acetabular roof defect on the right and demonstrates also the areas of ossification in the soft tissues laterally.

5.19 OA of the hip characterised principally by substantial subarticular radiolucencies ('geodes'). Note that these lesions are essentially in a superior polar position and contiguous across the joint space. Other features of OA are virtually absent. This has also been called 'cystic arthrosis' of the hip.

5.22

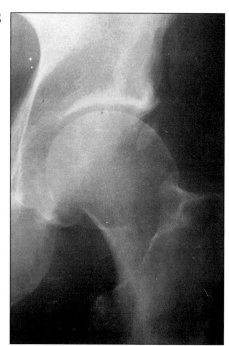

5.22 OA of the hip at an early stage of evolution. Note the slight superior joint space narrowing and also the area of radiolucency in the acetabular roof with, as yet, no evidence of an abnormality in the femoral head.

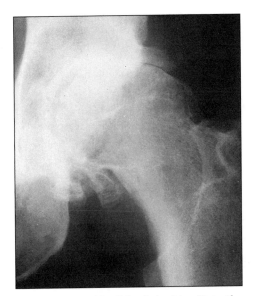 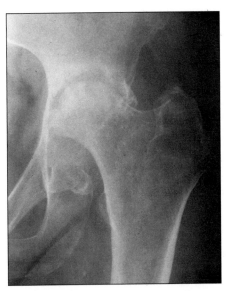

5.23 Hypertrophic OA of the hip. Note the abundant osteophytosis and relative absence of destructive features.

5.24 Atrophic OA of the hip. Severe destruction is demonstrated, involving principally the articular surfaces with ill-defined sclerosis. An apparently wide 'joint space' is shown. Note the absence of secondary bone response.

Erosive OA

An unequivocal erosive variant of OA occurs predominantly in the hands, involving the usual joints: terminal interphalangeal joints (TIPJs), proximal interphalangeal joints (PIPJs), and sometimes metacarpophalangeal joints (MCPJs) (Kidd and Peter, 1966). The main feature (**5.25**) is of disruption of the articular surface with frank loss of articular cortex, soft tissue swelling but seldom osteoporosis. The appearances may be quite bizarre at the point of greatest destruction (**5.26**) and are scintigraphically avidly abnormal (**5.27**, **5.28**), particularly during their evolution. However, careful comparison between patients with these radiological features and age/sex matched controls do not suggest a clinically distinctive subset, but rather the more aggressive end of the OA spectrum in the hand (Cobby *et al.*, 1990). Distinction between erosive OA and psoriatic arthropathy should not present a problem if the concept of the bare area and distribution of lesions is borne in mind (Martel *et al.*, 1980) (**5.29–5.31**). Psoriatic arthritis is essentially a disease of the synovium causing erosion and bone proliferation at the bare area, whereas OA is, by definition, a disease of the articular surfaces and subchondral bone (**5.32**).

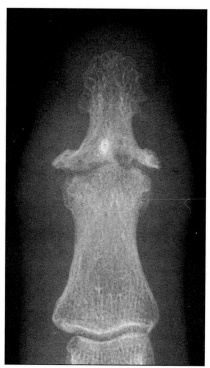

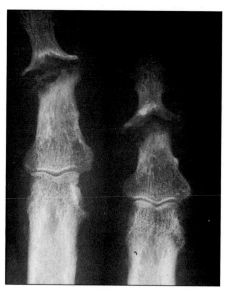

5.26 Erosive OA: gross appearances. Erosive disease is shown at the terminal interphalangeal joints of the ring and little fingers. The features are similar to those shown in **5.25**, but note a relatively wide 'joint space'.

5.25 Erosive OA in a terminal interphalangeal joint. The appearances are typical. There is soft tissue swelling, extensive destruction of the articular surfaces, ill-defined subchondral radiolucencies and obvious loss of bone.

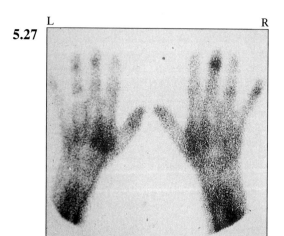

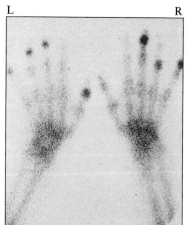

5.27, 5.28 Scintigraphic assessment in erosive OA (the same case as shown in **5.25**). Note on the blood pool image (**5.27**) considerably increased activity at the TIPJ of the middle finger on the right. A subsequent delayed image (**5.28**) confirms increased activity at this joint. Note also that many other TIPJs and PIPJs are scintigraphically abnormal. These, however, did not exhibit erosive features on plain film at the time of the scintigram.

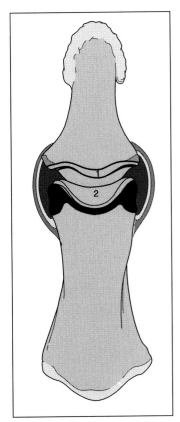

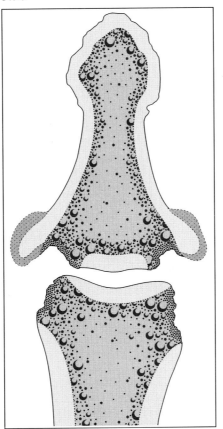

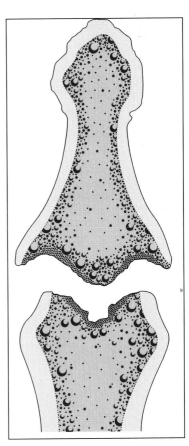

5.29 The concept of the bare area (from Martel, 1980). Articular surface diseases will involve those areas covered by cartilage (1 & 2), whereas synovial diseases such as rheumatoid disease and psoriasis will first manifest where synovium touches bone not covered by articular cartilage (black).

5.30, 5.31 The principal radiological differences are shown between psoriatic arthritis (**5.30**) and erosive OA (**5.31**) (after Martel, 1980). **5.30** New bone formation is shown in association with erosion of the bare areas. Note the normal articular surfaces. **5.31**. Here the predominant abnormality is on the articular surface and not at the bare area.

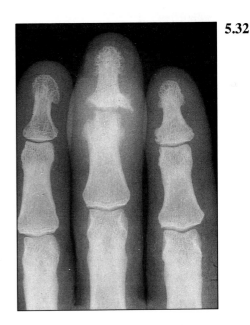

5.32 Psoriatic arthritis. Contrast these appearances with those shown in **5.25**. Note the major differences between erosive OA in **5.25** and these appearances as explained in **5.30** and **5.31**.

The role of crystals

Calcium pyrophosphate dihydrate (CPPD)

Radiological chondrocalcinosis is usually caused by CPPD and a normal age-related phenomenon peaking at about 40% in 80-year-olds (Wilkins *et al.*, 1983). The radiological features are typical, comprising linear or granular calcification in fibro- and hyaline cartilage, and hence occurring in those joints in which the former predominate (**5.33**). As the degree of deposition becomes gross, so chondrocalcinosis may be expected also at other joints, in the capsule and enthesis (**5.34**). When episodes of crystal-shedding associated with acute synovitis occur, radiology is generally unhelpful, apart from revealing a joint effusion. Over time chondrocalcinosis may come or go (**5.35**, **5.36**). It may be very ephemeral indeed (**5.37**, **5.38**)!

5.33

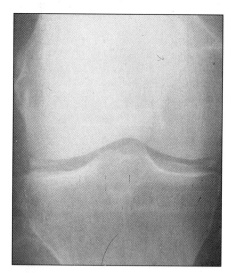

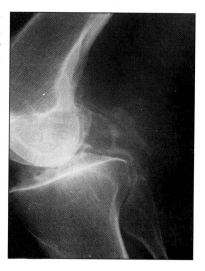

5.33 Chondrocalcinosis caused by pyrophosphate deposition at the knee. Typical linear and granular calcification is demonstrated in hyaline cartilage and the menisci.

5.34 A more gross example of chondrocalcinosis shows depositions also in the joint capsule and ligamentous structures dorsal to the knee.

5.35

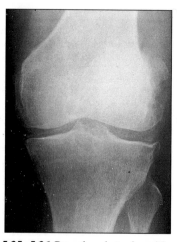

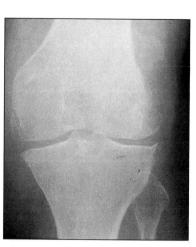

5.36

5.35, 5.36 Pyrophosphate deposition – crystal shedding. In **5.35** typical linear chondrocalcinosis is demonstrated involving both compartments. However, 2 years later (**5.36**), after several episodes of acute crystal arthritis, the chondrocalcinosis is no longer visible. Note also, however, that hyaline cartilage width has also been reduced.

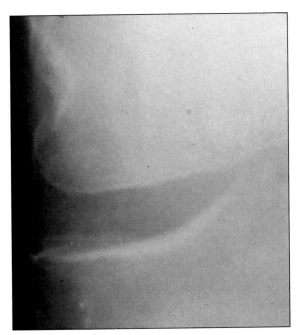 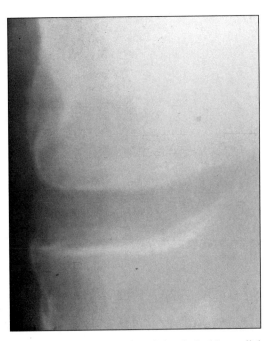

5.37, 5.38 Transient chondrocalcinosis. At the time of admission this man with chondrocalcinosis in his medial compartment (**5.37**) suffered an acute attack of crystal arthritis. Twenty-four hours later (**5.38**), the chondrocalcinosis is no longer visible.

Previously, there has been considerable confusion as to the relationship between chondrocalcinosis and a hypertrophic form of OA, termed 'pyrophosphate arthropathy'. The confusion was predominantly caused by the fact that no logical sequence occurred between the episodes of crystal-shedding, chondrocalcinosis and the development of a structural arthritis. Radiologically, some patients with classical 'pyrophosphate arthropathy' have been shown not to have pyrophosphate crystals either in capsule, synovium, cartilage or bone. The radiological variants of this subset have been studied at length (Resnick *et al.*, 1977), the major features being unusual joint involvement compared with ordinary OA, unusual intra-articular distribution, marked subchondral radiolucencies, osteophyte formation and occasional progression, destruction and fragmentation. Classical examples of the major hypertrophic form of OA are demonstrated (**5.39, 5.40**), as is the unusual intra-articular distribution, for example particularly involving the patellofemoral joint (**5.41, 5.42**). Subchondral radiolucencies may be marked (**5.43, 5.44**). Pyrophosphate arthropathy may be inferred when these features occur together in a given joint.

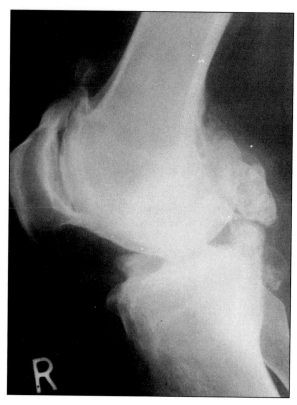

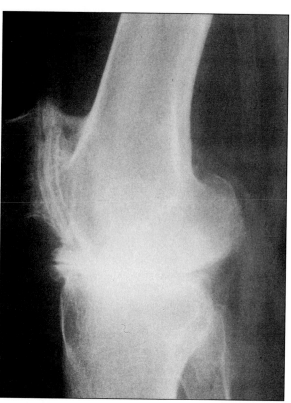

5.39, 5.40 Two examples of pyrophosphate arthropathy involving the knee. In **5.39** note the prolific new bone formation, particularly at the patellofemoral joint, with areas of separate though not loose ossification in the suprapatellar pouch and in the posterior joint space. Note the relative absence of any bone destruction or other major feature. This patient (**5.40**) with pyrophosphate modified rheumatoid disease shows no evidence whatever of rheumatoid arthritis. There is, however, abundant hypertrophic osteophytosis and joint space narrowing in all compartments particularly demonstrated at the patellofemoral joint.

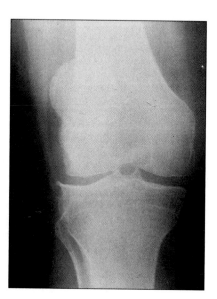

5.41, 5.42 Pyrophosphate arthropathy. Atypical intra-articular involvement. In this example the knee compartments are virtually normal save for minor osteophytosis laterally, whereas gross abnormality of the patellofemoral joint is demonstrated (**5.42**).

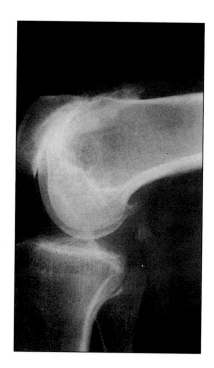

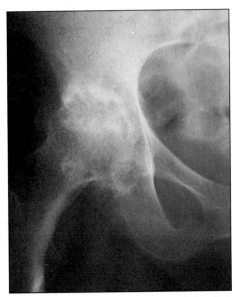

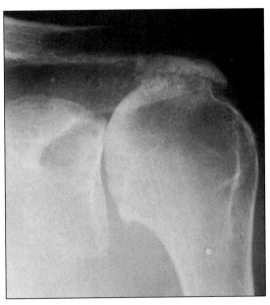

5.43 Pyrophosphate arthropathy – subchondral radiolucencies. Note the extensive abnormality of the contiguous areas of the superior polar region. Multiple 'cyst-like' radiolucencies are demonstrated with abundant adjacent sclerosis.

5.44 In this example of pyrophosphate arthropathy a complete rotator cuff tear is present. Consequently a pseudoarthrosis exists between the glenohumeral head and the undersurface of the acromion. Note the presence of multiple subchondral radiolucencies at this pseudoarthrosis together with the presence of sclerosis.

Calcium hydroxyapatite

Whilst, typically, deposition of hydroxyapatite is recognised in calcific periarthritis, recent work has shown that it is found in association with an atrophic destructive form of OA in the shoulder and knee (Dieppe *et al.*, 1984; McCarty *et al.*, 1981). The principal radiological features are those of considerable, progressive bone destruction in elderly, somewhat osteoporotic women with the absence of secondary bone response, and large joint effusions on plain film (**5.45**, **5.46**, **5.47**). The joints are markedly unstable. Radiologically, destructive OA of the hip shares the same characteristics, the appearances having been previously described as analgesic or 'Indocid' hip (**5.48**, **5.49**). The relationship between this form of destructive OA and non-steroidal anti-inflammatory agents has not been proven (Doherty *et al.*, 1986).

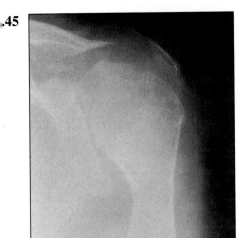

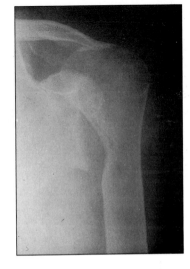

5.45 Destructive OA of the shoulder joint. Note the considerable bone destruction, excavation of the humeral neck, absence of osteophytosis and reactive sclerosis.

5.46 The same shoulder as shown in **5.45** but on this occasion in a relaxed position. The humeral head is now shown to have migrated up under the residual excavated acromioclavicular joint confirming that the rotator cuff is completely deficient.

5.47

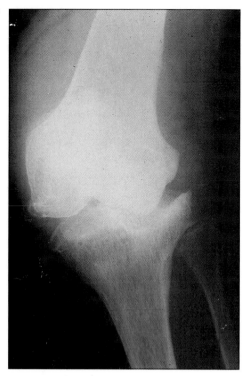

5.47 Destructive OA of the knee. A single AP view demonstrates a huge effusion in the suprapatellar pouch and destruction of the knee compartments without osteophytosis. Joint fluid was full of hydroxyapatite.

5.48

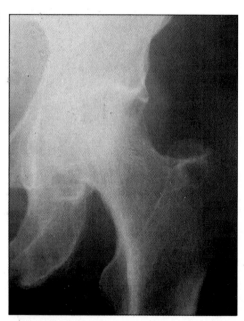

5.49

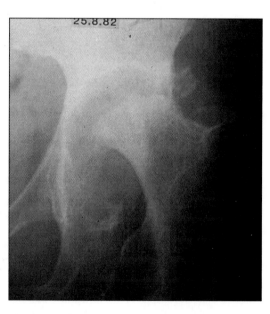

5.48, 5.49 Rapidly destructive hip OA. Also previously called analgesic or 'Indocid hip'. Note the progression from an essentially normal hip (**5.48**) to severe destructive OA (**5.49**). Note the similarity to erosive OA in the hands (**5.26**), insofar as the lesion predominantly involves the articular surfaces with a wide 'joint space'.

The role of cystals in OA has been reappraised in the light of recent work (Dieppe and Watt, 1985). The position is best summarised (**5.50**) as not proven, but the current most likely view is that an association exists between the deposition of pyrophosphate crystals and a hypertrophic bone response on one hand, and an atrophic bone response and hydroxyapatite crystals on the other. These are not seen as cause and effect, but rather as both caused by other unknown stem factors. It is important to remember that these are processes which may be transient, and that a hypertrophic form of disease may progress to an atrophic form (**5.51, 5.52**). Charcot-type arthropathy may be considered to fall at the extremes of these categories, with either markedly hypertrophic or atrophic changes (**5.53, 5.54**).

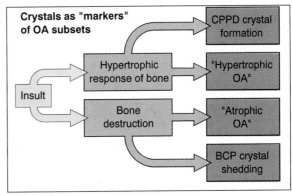

5.50 The most viable current concept of the relationships between crystals and OA.

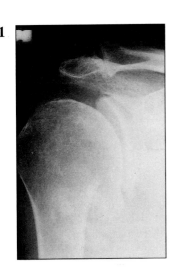

5.51, 5.52 This case illustrates the concept of disease processes rather than diseases themselves. This shoulder (**5.51**) demonstrates typical features of hypertrophic OA with abundant osteophytosis and intact articular surfaces. At the time of this radiograph the joint was full of pyrophosphate crystals. About 2 years later (**5.52**) severe destruction of the glenohumeral joint has occurred. The osteophyte has been destroyed. A joint effusion is now present in the subdeltoid bursa, the appearances now being typical of destructive OA. The joint at this time contained abundant hydroxyapatite in addition to a few pyrophosphate crystals. Clearly a major change has occurred within this joint but the processes involved are essentially unknown.

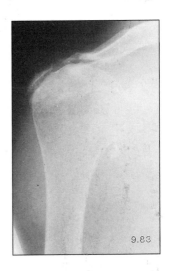

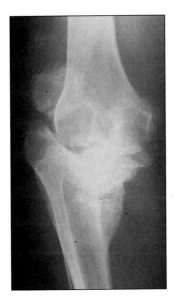

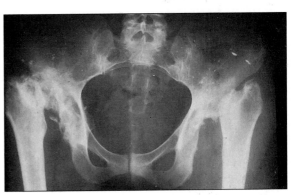

5.53, 5.54 Two examples of Charcot arthropathy. Essentially the appearances are those of rather gross OA with hypertrophic features dominating (**5.53**) and with bone destruction (**5.54**). Note in both instances the considerable deformity that has occurred, yet there is preserved bone density, indicating continued limb function.

Other clues to aetiology

Clearly some joints are at risk of developing OA by virtue of their morphology, for example following trauma or congenital dislocation of the hip (**5.55**). The fact that some joints might be 'dysplastic' has prompted a series of measurements to establish the normal range, for example, in the hip (**5.56**) (Murray, 1965). However, it is likely that these measurements are too crude to detect subtle abnormalities which are clearly visible on plain X-ray. Examples are shown in **5.57–5.60** of two patients who had avascular necrosis of the hip joint. Over a period of time the well-contained but avascular femoral head of the first patient showed little progression of OA, whereas in the other, partially uncovered femoral head, there was rapid progression. Similarly, at the knee dysplastic features have also been recognised (Cooke, 1985). In some patients, load line films clearly demonstrate an abnormal valgus angulation of the lower femur and/or varus angulation of the upper tibia (**5.61, 5.62**). These 'dysplastic' features may represent an evolutionary under-design of human joints rather than a dysplasia (*see* Chapter 8). Angular deformity of the joint may also place abnormal stress on adjacent bony structures; OA, pyrophosphate-associated arthropathy and rheumatoid disease all being associated with upper tibial stress fractures (**5.63**).

Even if the biological responses to the deranged

5.55

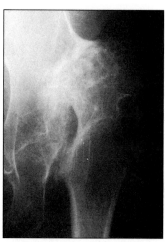

5.55 Congenital dislocation of the hip with obvious secondary degenerative arthritis. This hip is clearly dysplastic. The acetabulum has not moulded normally, indeed it is difficult to visualise where the acetabular fossa may have been originally.

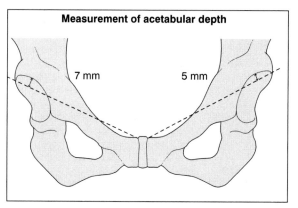

Measurement of acetabular depth

7 mm   5 mm

5.56

5.56 Normal acetabular depth. After the method advocated by Murray (1965), the normal acetabular depth should exceed 8mm.

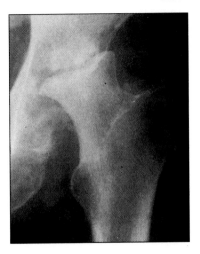
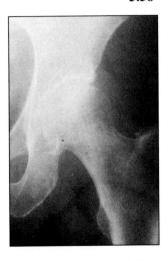
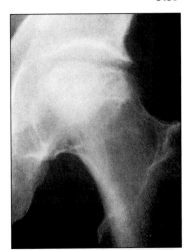

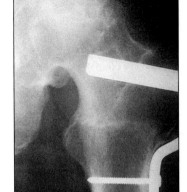

5.57–5.60 The role of acetabular/hip dysplasia on the development of OA. Two patients are shown with avascular necrosis of the femoral head. In **5.57** the patient has a normally moulded acetabulum with a well-covered femoral head. In **5.58** a patient who subsequently developed rapidly progressing OA has a shallow acetabulum with a partly uncovered femoral head. In **5.59**, 5 years later, and following a McMurray osteotomy, the first patient's hip shows virtually no evidence of disease progression, whereas in **5.60**, which shows the femoral head only 2 years later, there is gross progression.

5.61 The concepts of lower femoral valgus dysplasia and other tibial varus angulation are demonstrated (Cooke, 1985).

5.62 An example of a load line film in a patient with dysplastic knees. Notice that although there is obvious varus angulation, the deformity occurs in the upper tibia and to some extent, in the lower tibia and lower femora.

5.61 **5.62** **5.63**

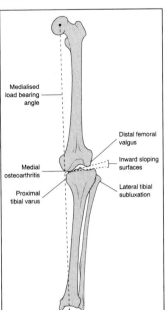
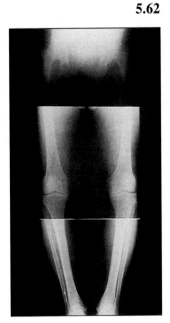
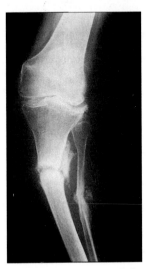

5.63 Stress fractures of the proximal tibia and fibula in association with valgus angulation caused by OA.

joint are understood, which they are not, other aetiological factors remain unknown. For example, a shortened femoral neck and large femoral head on the right in the patient shown in **5.64–5.67**, who had previously had a juvenile synovitis, might be deemed to predispose that joint to OA. In the outcome it was the normal contralateral hip which showed the disease. Hence other sensitive imaging modalities may be necessary to capture and understand the evolution of OA.

5.64

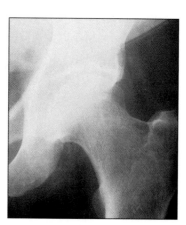

5.65

5.66

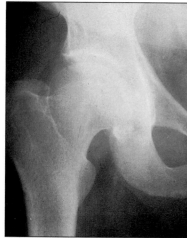

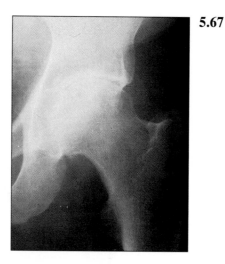

5.67

5.64–5.67 In spite of a pre-existing abnormal right hip caused by juvenile arthritis, it is the apparently normal left hip which 3 years later develops features of OA.

Scintigraphy

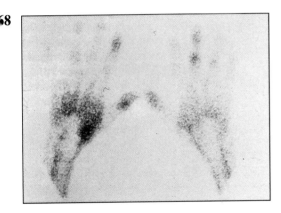

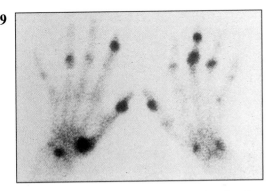

The [99m]technetium labelled diphosphonate bone scanning agents have been known to be very sensitive to the presence of OA for some years (Thomas *et al.*, 1975). Individual abnormal joints present intense foci of localised abnormal activity on the delayed phase of the radionuclide scintigram (**5.68, 5.69**). The degree and extent of abnormality on the perfusion or blood pool phase is thought to parallel the degree of inflammation and synovial disease (*see* **5.25, 5.27, 5.28**). Scintigraphy, however, has introduced the possibility of osteophyte in OA being biologically inert (**5.70–5.72**). What seems to be happening is that abnormal scintigraphic activity occurs, evolves and regresses before plain film radiographic changes are apparent (**5.73–5.77**). Indeed, the presence of abnormal activity on a scintigram is highly predictive of subsequent skeletal change but not vice versa (Hutton *et al.*, 1986). Scintigraphy has also taught us that OA, rather than being perceived as a polyarticular disease, may in effect be a 'monarthritis multiplex'. Data from scintigraphy of the knee joint also indicate that OA is scintigraphically not a homogeneous condition (McCrae *et al.*, 1987). Four major subsets have been identified, each carrying correspondingly different radiographic correlates (**5.78, Table 5.2**). For example, tramline activity seems closely allied to rim osteophytosis and not particularly to joint space narrowing or subchondral sclerosis (**5.79, 5.80**), whereas the extended pattern is thought to be prognostically more significant, and associated with bone attrition and sclerosis (**5.81, 5.82**).

5.68, 5.69 Skeletal scintigraphy using [99m]technetium labelled HMDP in hand OA. Note the intense localised foci of increased activity at typically involved joints in the delayed phase image (**5.69**). Most osteoarthritic joints are not particularly abnormal on the earlier blood pool image (**5.68**).

5.71

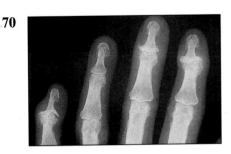

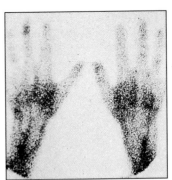

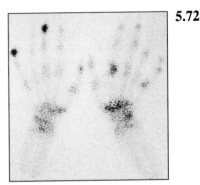

5.72

5.70–5.72 A disparity exists between the radiographic (**5.70**) and scintigraphic (**5.71, 5.72**) features of hand OA in this patient. Note the radiograph reveals typical TIPJ OA in three joints, whereas the scintigram, both on early (**5.71**) and delayed (**5.72**) images demonstrates that only two of these joints are scintigraphically active. This implies that the osteophytosis and other features shown of the index finger TIPJ on the radiograph were biologically inert. The joint may, therefore, be perceived to be stable and 'healed'.

5.73

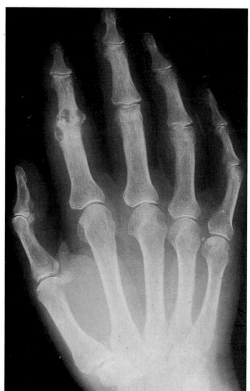

5.74

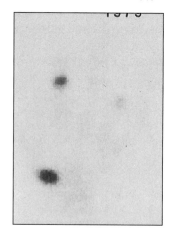

5.7

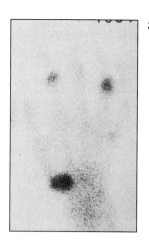

5.76

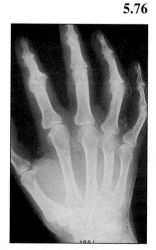

5.7

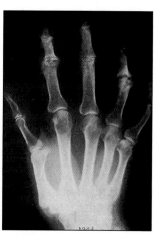

5.73–5.77 Scintigraphic and radiographic evolution of erosive OA in the hand. These images demonstrate that scintigraphy predicts subsequent radiographic change. In 1979 (**5.73**) a hand radiograph demonstrates erosive OA of the index finger PIPJ, no other abnormality being seen. However, a scintigram in 1979 (**5.74, 5.75**) demonstrates not only obvious activity at this joint but also at the thumb CMCJ and, though much less marked, at the PIPJ of the ring finger. A subsequent scintigram in 1981 demonstrated regression of the abnormality at the index PIPJ, further increased activity at the thumb CMCJ and also at the ring PIPJ. The radiographs in 1981 (**5.76**) and subsequently in 1984 (**5.77**), demonstrate the progression of change at the index PIPJ and the unequivocal evolution of aggressive OA at the thumb CMCJ and ring PIPJ.

5.78

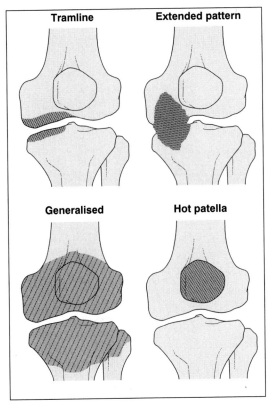

Tramline   Extended pattern

Generalised   Hot patella

5.78 A schematic drawing of the four types of abnormal scintigraphy findings at the knee joint in OA (after McCrae *et al.*, 1987; McCrae *et al.*, 1992).

Table 5.2 The principal characteristics of the scintigraphic subsets of knee OA (after McCrae *et al.*, 1987; McCrae *et al.*, 1992).

'Tramline'	
	Uptake at the joint margin.
	May be in one compartment only.
	Best seen on late (bone) image.
	May reflect active osteophytosis
'Generalised'	
	Uptake all around the knee joint.
	Seen on early and late phases.
	Clears after i. a. steroids.
	May reflect synovitis.
'Extended'	
	Isotope extends away from joint line.
	May be in one compartment only.
	Best seen on late (bone) image.
	May reflect changing subchondral bone.
'Hot patella'	
	Uptake in the patella only.
	A frequent, often isolated pattern.
	Significance uncertain.

5.79

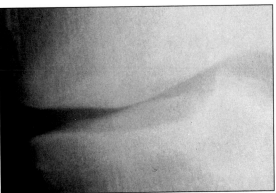

5.80

5.79, 5.80 Radiographic correlation of tramline activity. The scintigram (**5.79**) demonstrates linear areas of increased activity separated by a 'joint space'. The radiograph **5.80** demonstrates rim osteophytosis, preserved joint space width and minimal subarticular sclerosis.

5.81

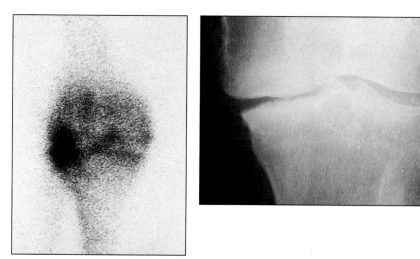

5.82

5.81, 5.82 Examples of the extended pattern in knee OA. A scintigram (**5.81**) demonstrates the increase in activity extending away from the articular surfaces. Radiographically (**5.82**), this corresponds to quite extensive and diffuse subchondral sclerosis.

Some data demonstrates that it is possible to suppress the inflammatory component of OA as demonstrated by a scintigram, using either intra-articular steroid (**5.83–5.86**), yttrium or NSAIDs, but that no change in the underlying bony pattern of OA occurs (**5.87–5.90**) (McCrae *et al.*, 1989). Long-term follow-up studies in knee OA demonstrate very little change radiographically or scintigraphically over a two-year period. There is, however, good correlation between symptomatology and scintigraphic abnormality (McCrae *et al.*, 1992).

5.83

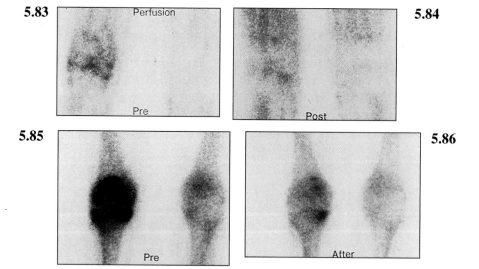

5.84

5.85

5.86

5.83–5.86 The effect of intra-articular steroid on scintigraphy in rheumatoid disease of the knee. **5.83, 5.84** Perfusion images before and after intra-articular steroid. **5.85, 5.86** Delayed images demonstrate a considerable suppression of abnormal activity two weeks after intra-articular steroid therapy. Note the main effect is on the blood pool image and the generalised activity on the delayed image.

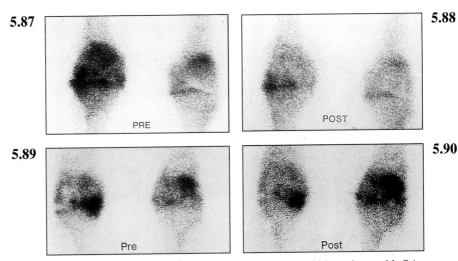

5.87 **5.88**

5.89 **5.90**

5.87–5.90 Similar images following intra-articular steroid in patients with OA. **5.87, 5.88** A patient with rather active synovitis in the right knee is shown to have appreciable suppression of generalised activity following steroid therapy. However, most of the joint line activity still remains, although this, too, is less than before. **5.89, 5.90** A patient with more conventional OA of the knee shows virtually no effect following intra-articular steroid therapy.

Magnetic resonance imaging (MRI)

Undoubtedly the newest and most exciting imaging modality to be relevant in OA is magnetic resonance imaging (MRI). Initially, attention was focused on the role of MRI in detecting focal pathology in joints, in particular meniscal tears (**5.91**), but also osteochondritis dissecans (**5.92**), avascular necrosis and many other conditions (Munk *et al.*, 1989). Careful post mortem work has demonstrated that MRI can demonstrate discrete defects in hyaline cartilage with and without the necessity of intra-articular contrast medium (Gylys-Morin *et al.*, 1987; Reiser *et al.*, 1988) (**5.93–5.96**). Estimation of actual T1 and T2 values for the deep and superficial layers of hyaline cartilage is also possible (Lehner *et al.*, 1989). These reflect the hydration level of the proteoglycans within the layers of cartilage and effect of the collagen network and it is possible to demonstrate these on images (**5.97, Table 5.3**). Confirmatory work in induced arthritis in dogs has also shown the earlier phase of cartilage swelling and over-hydration (**5.98, 5.99**) following anterior cruciate ligament transection (Brawnstein *et al.*, 1990).

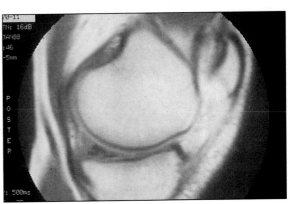

5.91

5.91 Magnetic resonance imaging – a medial meniscal tear. An obvious tear of the posterior horn of the medial meniscus is demonstrated on proton density (mixed T_1W–T_2W) image. Note the high signal (white) lines extending through the otherwise low signal (black) posterior horn of the medial meniscus. Note how also hyaline cartilage is beautifully demonstrated (grey), articular cortex being low signal (black).

5.92

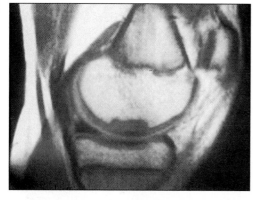

5.92 An example of osteochondritis dissecans of the medial femoral condyle. Notice a low signal (black) abnormality at the apex of the condyle with slight swelling of the overlying hyaline cartilage.

5.93

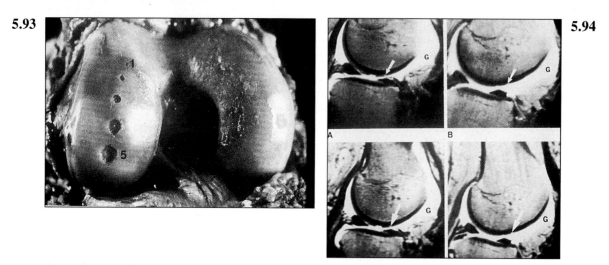

5.94

5.93, 5.94 Magnetic resonance imaging (MRI) demonstrates iatrogenic defects in hyaline cartilage in post-mortem specimens (from Gylys-Morten *et al.*, 1987). The specimen in **5.93** shows defects drilled in the medial femoral condyle. Subsequent MR images (**5.94**) in which intra-articular contrast medium (gadolinium) has been injected. Note the ease with which the defects can be demonstrated on the MR images.

5.95

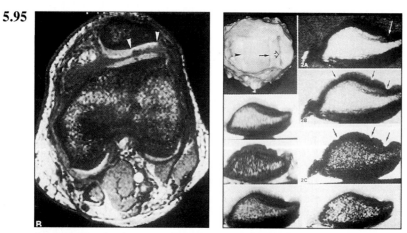

5.96

5.95, 5.96 Studies in chondromalacia of the patellae (from Reiser *et al.*, 1988) demonstrate obvious defects in the lateral articular facet of the patella (**5.95**). Subsequent images of the excised patella using various pulse sequences demonstrate unequivocally the defects in hyaline cartilage. The reader is referred to the original article for further detail.

5.97, Table 5.3 Magnetic resonance imaging in hyaline cartilage disease. **5.97** Abnormal hyaline cartilage is demonstrated (top left). Subsequent images demonstrate increased signal caused by overhydration (white) and areas of abnormality low signal (black) associated with change in deep layers of hyaline cartilage.

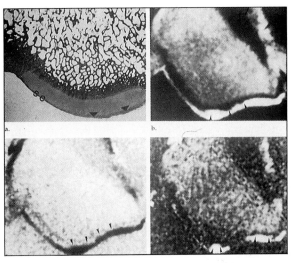

Table 5.3 Measurements of the characteristics of hyaline cartilage layers at MR imaging demonstrate that measureable differences can be recorded *in vivo*. (From Lehner *et al.*, 1989.)

Layer	Water content (% of Wet Weight) (n = 9)	T1 (msec) (n = 9)	T2 (msec) (n = 9)	Layer Thickness (mm) (n = 23)
	Mean ± Standard Error			
Superficial	82 ± 3	580 ± 65	77 ± 20	1.4 ± 0.5
Deep	76 ± 3	350 ± 35	51 ± 15	2.2 ± 1.3*

* Epiphyseal cartilage included

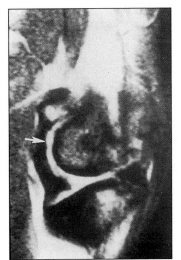

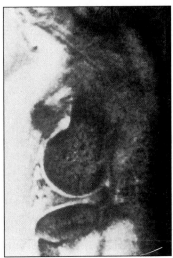

5.98, 5.99 MR imaging in a dog knee following an anterior cruciate resection demonstrates considerable increase in hyaline cartilage thickness on the operated knee (left) compared with the unoperated knee (right) (from Brawnstein *et al.*, 1990).

In practical clinical applications, however, it is possible to demonstrate abnormal cartilage signal and thickness (**5.100, 5.101**) but frequently the disease process has advanced beyond that stage by the time patients are imaged (**5.102, 5.103**). Other new features on MRI in OA have been established, however (McAlindon *et al.*, 1991). These include the obvious displacement and attrition of menisci, para-articular cystic or ganglion-like lesions and variable osteophytosis, the most strikingly interesting of which is the so-called 'bright osteophyte' thought to represent freshly deposited bone and possibly corresponding to the tramline activity seen on skeletal scintigraphy (**5.104, 5.105**) (McAlindon *et al.*, 1989). Differences between the subchondral cystic lesions have also been observed, some apparently containing essentially a watery content, others a high lipid value (**5.106, 5.107**).

5.100
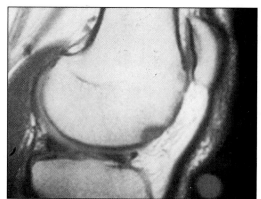
5.101
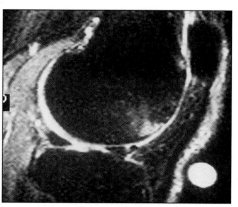

5.100, 5.101 Sagittal MR images in OA demonstrate abnormal hyaline cartilage thinning and subchondral bony response in a proton density (mixed T_1W–T_2W) image (**5.100**), and a STIR (short tau inversion recovery) image (**5.101**). Note hyaline cartilage thinning at the apex of the femoral condyle. Immediately dorsal to this on the STIR sequence particularly, one can see low signal in thickened hyaline cartilage similar to the abnormalities shown in **5.95**. Areas of increased signal on the STIR sequence anteriorly in the femoral condyle suggest increased fluid content and marrow oedema.

5.102
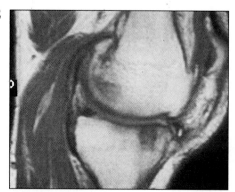
5.103
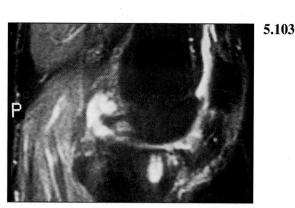

5.102, 5.103 Advanced OA of the knee. Sagittal MR images in the proton density (mixed T_1W–T_2W) (**5.102**) and STIR sequences (**5.103**) demonstrate advanced disease. In addition to obvious thinning of hyaline cartilage with joint effusion, particularly apparent in the suprapatellar pouch, extensive subchondral abnormalities are shown with a cyst in the upper tibia anteriorly. The cartilage is so badly destroyed that no particular measureable characteristic can be determined.

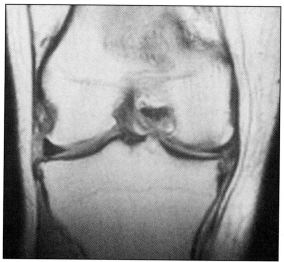

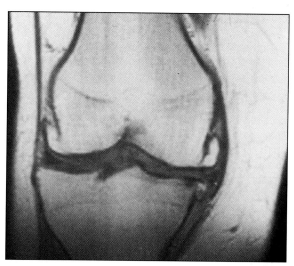

5.104 Coronal MR image (proton density mixed T_1W–T_2W image) demonstrates other features in OA. The medial meniscus is grossly abnormal and extruded medially from the joint line. High signal within and adjacent to it suggests some cystic degeneration deep to the medial collateral ligament. There is some hyaline cartilage thinning over the medial condyle and reduced subchondral signal. Note that the medial joint line shows osteophytosis, the marrow of which shows increased signal and is 'bright'.

5.105 An even more gross example of rim osteophytosis with 'bright' signal in the marrow of osteophyte.

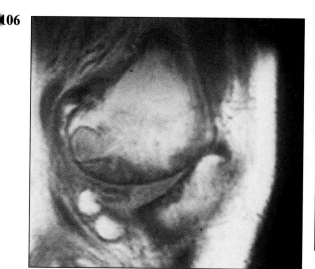

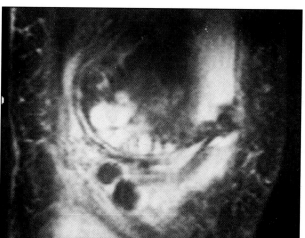

5.106, 5.107 At least two types of 'cystic' lesion are demonstrated in knee OA. A proton density (mixed T_1W–T_2W) (**5.106**) and a STIR sequence (**5.107**) demonstrate cystic lesions in the femoral condyle which are low signal on proton density but high signal on the STIR sequence. The converse occurs in the lesions in the tibia. The implication is that the femoral lesions contain a high water content, whereas those in the tibia contain high lipid.

Summary

Radiologically, OA is a heterogeneous group of disorders, possibly with a common end point of joint failure. It is always important to remember that radiology, by any technique, does not demonstrate pain, and occasional complete misinterpretations of radiographic images can result (**5.108**, **5.109**). It is important to emphasise that radiologically OA is not a one-way disease progression. Even over a long time span the features of the disease wax and wane (Masardo *et al.*, 1988). Joint failure is not inevitable and unequivocal healing does occur. The skeleton is capable of abundant bone formation (**5.110**) and even reconstitution of articular surfaces and joint space width (**5.111**, **5.112**). Regression may also be demonstrated scintigraphically (**5.113**, **5.114**). Careful analysis of the radiological features suggests a concept akin to a stability loop (**5.115**). Normal joints are rendered unstable by a series of factors, only some of which are known, but which clearly include trauma, ageing, under-design and inflammatory processes. Diagnostic imaging is capable of demonstrating the response to this instability with the formation of osteophyte and subchondral bone change and recognises a spectrum of those responses. Scintigraphy, and perhaps MRI, can show change before structural abnormality occurs. What processes these changes represent, what pathological processes are involved, and what therapeutic manipulations are possible are entirely unknown. The nature of those processes is the outstanding clinical, biochemical and radiological challenge in this group of disorders.

5.108

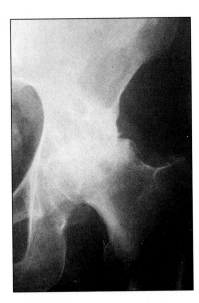

5.109

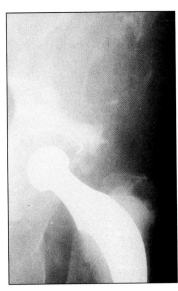

5.108, 5.109 Radiographs do not demonstrate pain. A patient with obvious superior polar OA (**5.108**) has an ill-defined radiolucency in the iliac crest above the acetabulum. This was, however, not noted and subsequent films at follow-up (**5.109**) show that this lesion is now a large destructive abnormality. This was shown later to be caused by a metastasis from renal cell carcinoma.

5.110

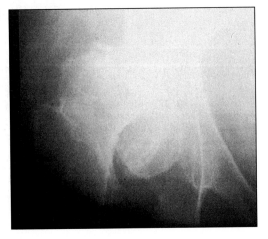

5.110 Abundant osteophytosis indicates the ability of this joint organ to respond to deranged anatomy although there is considerable superolateral migration. Note the huge osteophyte that has developed inferomedial to the femoral head and neck in an attempt to reconstruct the major weight-bearing surface of the femoral head itself.

5.111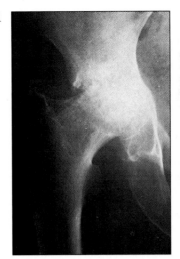
5.112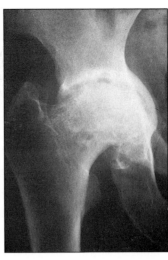

5.111, 5.112 Healing in acute OA. **5.111** demonstrates severe destructive OA with bone attrition, total loss of joint space width and extensive subchondral bone destruction. Some time later articular surfaces have reappeared and a joint space has been re-established. Whilst this is obviously not a normal hip, there is clear evidence of damage limitation and healing.

5.113, 5.114 Evidence of scintigraphic regression of OA in the knee. Obvious diminution in abnormal activity has occurred between 1986 and 1987. Note that not only is generalised activity reduced but also the tramline activity associated with rim osteophytosis. The patient had symptomatically improved at follow-up.

5.113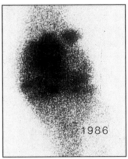
5.114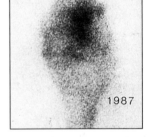

5.115 A stability loop represents a simple management concept. It suggests that a stable joint is rendered abnormal by processes unknown. The resulting instability evokes a response which will tend to recreate a state of stability even though this may not be identical to the original position. It may be argued that the creation of instability in OA is only partially understood, trauma and evolutionary under-design being two possible factors. Osteoarthritis, as it is recognised, represents responses to these changes. These responses are clearly very varied and themselves only partially understood.

5.115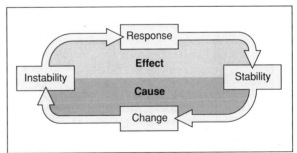

References and further reading

Brawnstein, E.M., Brandt, K.D., Albrecht, M. (1990) MRI demonstration of hypertrophic articular cartilage repair in osteoarthritis. *Skeletal Radiol.* **19**, 335–339.

Cobby, M., Watt, I., Dieppe, P. (1989) *Imaging in osteoarthritis.* Russell, R.G.G., Dieppe, P. (Eds.) Osteoarthritis: current research and prospects for pharmacological intervention. IBC, London.

Cobby, M., Cushnaghan, J., Creamer, P., Dieppe, P., Watt, I. (1990) Erosive osteoarthritis: is it a separate disease entity? *Clinical Radiol.* **42**, (258–263).

Cooke, T.D.V. (1985) Pathogenic mechanisms in polyarticular osteoarthritis. *Clin. Rheum. Dis.*, **11**, 203–210.

Dieppe, P.A., Doherty, M., Macfarlane, D.G., Hutton, C.W. *et al.* (1984) Apatite associated destructive arthritis. *Br. J. Rheumatol.*, **23**, 84–91.

Dieppe, P., Watt, I. (1985) Crystal deposition in osteoarthritis: an opportunistic event? *Clin. Rheum. Dis.*, **11**, 367–392.

Doherty, M., Holt, M., MacMillan, P., Watt, I., Dieppe, P. (1986) A re-appraisal of 'analgesic hip'. *Br. J. Rheumatol.*, **45**, 272–276.

Gibson, P.H., Goodfellow, J.W. (1986) Stress radiography in degenerative arthritis of the knee. *J. Bone Joint Surgery*, **68B**, 608–609.

Gylys-Morin, D.M., Hajek, P.C., Sartoris, D.J., Resnick, D. (1987) Articular cartilage defects: detectability in cadaver knees with MR. *Am. J. Roentgenology*, **148**, 1153–1157.

Hall, F.M., Wyshack, G. (1980) Thickness of articular cartilage in the normal knee. *J. Bone Joint Surg.*, **62A**, 508–513.

Hutton, C.W., Higgs, E.R., Jackson, P.C., Watt, I., Dieppe, P.A. (1986) [99m] technetium HMDP bone scanning generalised nodal osteoarthritis – a four hour bone scan image predicts radiographic change. *Annals of the Rheumatic Diseases*, **45**, 622–626.

Kellgren, J.H., Lawrence, J.S. (1957) Radiological assessment of osteoarthrosis. *Ann. Rheum. Dis.*, **16**, 494–502.

Kidd, L.K., Peter, J.B. (1966) Erosive osteoarthritis. *Radiology*, **86**, 640–647.

Leach, R.E., Gregg, T., Siber, F.J. (1970) Weight-bearing radiography in osteoarthritis of the knee. *Radiology*, **97**, 265–268.

Lehner, K.B., Rechl, H.P., Gmeinwieser, J.K., Heuck, A.F. *et al.* (1989) Structure, function and degeneration of bovine hyaline cartilage: assessment with MR imaging in vitro. *Radiology*, **170**, 495–499.

Makela, P., Virtama, P., Dean, P.B. (1979) Finger joint swelling: correlation with age, gender and manual labour. *Am. J. Roentgenology*, **132**, 939–943.

Martel, W., Stuck, K.J., Dworin, A.M., Hyland, R.G. (1980) Erosive osteoarthritis and psoriatic arthritis: a radiologic comparison in the hand, wrist and foot. *Am. J. Roentgenology*, **134**, 125–135.

Masardo, L., Watt, I., Cushnaghan, J., Dieppe, P. (1988) An eight year prospective study of established peripheral joint osteoarthritis. *Br. J. Rheumatol.*, **27**, 63 (Abstract).

McCarty, D.J., Cheung, H.S., Halverson, P.B., Garancis, J.C. (1981) 'Milwaukee shoulder syndrome'. microspherules containing hydroxyapatite, active collagenase and neutral protease in patients with rotator cuff defects and glenohumeral osteoarthritis. *Sem. Arthritis Rheum.*, **11**(suppl. 1), 119–121.

McAlindon, T.E., Watt, I., McCrae, F., Goddard, P., Dieppe, P. (1991) Magnetic resonance imaging in osteoarthritis of the knee: correlation with radiographic and scintigraphic findings. *Ann. Rheum. Dis.*, 50, 14–20.

McAlindon, T.E., McCrae, F., Watt, I., Dieppe, P.A. (1989) Correlation between scintigraphic patterns of magnetic resonance images in osteoarthritis of the knee. *Br. J. Rheumatol.*, **28**(suppl. 2), 8(Abstract).

McCrae, F., Shouls, J., Dieppe, P., Watt, I. (1987) Heterogeneity of osteoarthritis of the knee. *Br. J. Rheumatol.*, **26**(suppl. 1), 45(Abstract).

McCrae, F., Palmer, M., Shouls, J., Watt, I., Dieppe, P. (1989) Scintigraphic assessment of synovial and bone responses after intra-articular [90]yttrium therapy. *Br. J. Rheumatol.*, **27**(suppl. 1), 13(Abstract).

McCrae, F., Shouls, J., Dieppe, P., Watt, I. The scintigraphic assessment of osteoarthritis of the knee joint. (1992). *Ann. Rheum. Dis.*, 51, 938–942.

Munk, P.L., Helms, C.A., Genant, H.K., Holt, R.G. (1989) Magnetic resonance imaging of the knee: current status, new directions. *Skeletal Radiol.*, **18**, 569–577.

Murray, R.O. (1965) Aetiology of primary osteoarthritis of the hip. *Br. J. Radiol.*, **38**, 810–824.

Reiser, M.F., Bongar, T.Z.G., Erlemann, R., Strobe, L.M. *et al.* (1988) Magnetic resonance in cartilaginous lesions of the knee joint with three-dimensional gradient-echo imaging. *Skeletal Radiol.*, **17**, 465–471.

Resnick, D., Niwayama, G., Joergen, T.G., Utsinger, P. *et al.* (1977) Clinical, radiographic and pathological abnormalities in calcium pyrophosphate deposition disease (CPPD): pseudogout. *Radiology*, **122**, 1–15.

Rogers, J., Watt, I., Dieppe, P. (1990) Comparison of visual and radiographic detection of bony changes at the knee joint. *Br. Med. J.*, **300**, 367–368.

Rosenberg, T.D., Paulos, L.E., Parker, R.D., Coward, D.B., Scott, S.M. (1988) The 45 degree postero-anterior flexion weight-bearing radiograph of the knee. *J. Bone Joint Surg.*, **70A**, 1479–1482.

Thomas, R.H., Resnick, D., Alazraki, N.P. (1975) Compartmental evaluation of osteoarthritis of the knee. A comparative study of available diagnostic modalities. *Radiology*, **116**, 858–864.

Wilkins, E., Dieppe, P., Maddison, P., Edison, G. (1983) Osteoarthritis and articular chondrocalcinosis in the elderly. *Ann. Rheum. Dis.*, **42**, 280–284.

6. Synovial Fluid Analysis

Paul Halverson

Synovial fluid, the viscous fluid found within the joint space, is a dialysate of plasma. Its viscosity derives from hyaluronate, a glycosaminoglycan secreted by type B synovioctyes which line the non-cartilaginous surface of the inside of the joint. Normally present in only small amounts, the volume of synovial fluid is variably increased in osteoarthritis (OA) and other types of arthritis. Excessive fluid accumulations (joint effusions) may occur in any joint but are most readily appreciated in the knee. Fluid is usually easily obtained from an effused joint by needle aspiration. Examination of the synovial fluid provides useful information about the arthropathy which caused it to form.

Handling of synovial fluid

Synovial fluid collected by needle and syringe should be transferred to a heparinised tube to prevent clotting. The study of synovial fluid in various arthropathies has been discussed extensively elsewhere (McCarty, 1993).

In OA, the fluid is viscous because of the qualitatively normal hyaluronate. This may be demonstrated by the so-called 'string sign' (6.1). As the needle is removed from the syringe, a drop of synovial fluid is expressed. If the column of fluid forms a string before breaking, normal viscosity is present. Alternatively, the integrity of the hyaluronate may be assessed by the mucin clot test (Ropes and Bauer, 1953). A few drops of 2% acetic acid are added to a few mls of synovial fluid in a test tube. A 'good' mucin clot describes the formation of a tight ropey precipitate in the bottom of the tube (6.2). 'Fair' or 'poor' mucin clot refers to an increasingly flocculent precipitate and is likely to be found in 'inflammatory' arthropathies.

6.1

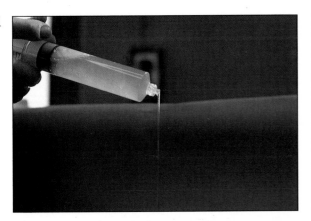

6.1 The 'string' sign. Viscous synovial fluid forms a string rather than individual drops when expressed from a syringe.

6.2

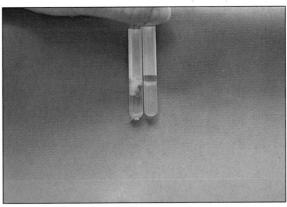

6.2 The mucin clot test. After addition of acetic acid, the osteoarthritic synovial fluid on the left forms a tight clot whereas the inflammatory fluid on the right forms a flocculent precipitate.

The synovial fluid leucocyte count is routinely performed with a haemocytometer and a differential white cell count may be obtained from a Wright's stained smear of synovial fluid. Synovial fluid leucocyte counts in OA (ordinarily <2,000/mm³) are referred to as 'non-inflammatory', although they exceed the number found in the fluid from completely normal joints. The higher leucocyte counts may reflect a low-grade inflammatory process in the osteoarthritic joint. The differential count shows a predominance of mononuclear cell types. This is in contrast to 'inflammatory' arthropathies in which the synovial fluid leucocyte count exceeds 2,000/mm³ and the differential count usually shows greater than 75% polymorphonuclear leucocytes.

A partial list of other arthropathies with synovial fluid characteristics similar to OA includes traumatic arthritis, internal derangement within the joint, such as a meniscal tear, avascular necrosis, Paget's disease of bone, Charcot's arthropathy, hypertrophic pulmonary osteoarthropathy, sympathetic effusions related to nearby extra-articular processes, and occasionally some arthropathies usually considered inflammatory which in the treated or resolving state may have 'non-inflammatory' features.

Polarised light microscopy (with phase contrast if possible) should be performed on a wet preparation of fresh synovial fluid. In OA, the fluid is clear with only a few mononuclear cells seen. Small amounts of debris consisting of cartilage fragments may be observed (**6.3, 6.4**).

In some cases weakly positively birefringent rhomboidal-shaped crystals may be seen. Usually these calcium pyrophosphate dihydrate (CPPD) crystals will be found in association with radiographically apparent chondrocalcinosis of hyaline or fibrocartilages.

Basic calcium phosphate (BCP) crystals are also known to be present in 30 to 60% of cases with OA (Dieppe *et al.*, 1979; Gibilisco *et al.*, 1985; Halverson *et al.*, 1986). BCP crystals are usually not detected by polarised light microscopy because these tiny crystals with an average length of about 0.1 µm are too small to be resolved by the light microscope. They do tend to aggregate into much larger masses but are not birefringent. They usually appear as debris but occasionally large crystal masses will appear as 'shiny coins' (**6.5**) (McCarty and Gatter, 1966).

6.3 Light micrograph of debris found in OA synovial fluid (× 400).

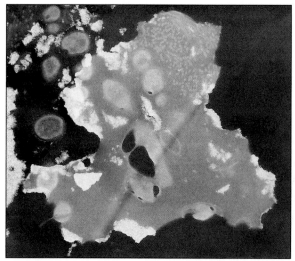

6.4 Electron micrograph of a synovial fluid pellet showing collagen fibres with characteristic banding. Basic calcium phosphate (BCP) crystals are also seen (× 10,600).

6.5 Phase contrast micrograph showing refractile BCP particles similar to 'shiny coins' (× 400).

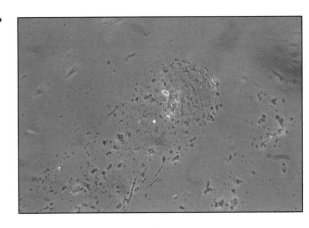

Additional methods of evaluating synovial fluid in OA

The calcium stain, alizarin red S, has been used by some to identify BCP crystals (Paul *et al.*, 1983). Only strong staining should be considered as suggestive (**6.6**). Unfortunately, this sensitive technique probably lacks sufficient specificity to be used in other than a screening capacity without additional confirmatory testing (Bardin *et al.*, 1987; Gordon *et al.*, 1989).

BCP crystals have been semi-quantitatively measured by binding of ^{14}C-labelled ethane-1-hydroxy-1, 1-diphosphonate (EHDP) (Halverson and McCarty, 1979). This diphosphonate, like other bone scanning agents, binds directly to BCP crystals from synovial fluid pellets resuspended in phosphate buffered saline. The method is sensitive to approximately 2 µg/ml of standard hydroxyapatite.

Both scanning and transmission electron microscopy with X-ray energy dispersive analysis satisfactorily identify BCP crystals. By transmission electron microscopy, individual crystals appear as short needles or rods usually not more than 0.1 µm in length (**6.7**). Plate-like crystals are more suggestive of octacalcium phosphate (**6.8**). Aggregated crystals are found in large masses embedded in a matrix (Cherian and Schumacher, 1982). By scanning electron microscopy, these masses appear as microspheroids approximately 2–20 µm in diameter (**6.9**). X-ray energy dispersive analysis reveals calcium to phosphorus molar ratios from 1.3–1.7. This range of values is explained by the fact that BCP crystals represent mixtures of partially carbonate-substituted hydroxyapatite (Ca:P=1.66), octacalcium phosphate (Ca:P=1.3), and rarely tricalcium phosphate (Ca:P=1.5) as demonstrated by Fourier transform infrared spectroscopy (McCarty *et al.*, 1983).

X-ray diffraction has also been used but requires a larger crystal specimen than electron microscopy. Recently, atomic force microscopy (AFM) has been successfully applied to the identification of synovial fluid microcrystals (Blair *et al.*, 1992).

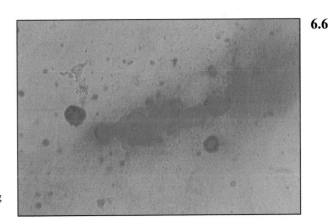

6.6 Alizarin red S preparation of synovial fluid containing BCP crystals showing strongly positive staining (× 400).

117

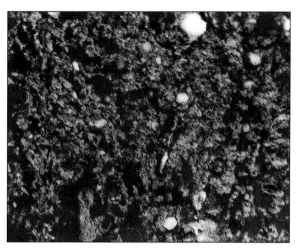

6.7 Electron micrograph of a synovial fluid pellet from a patient with BCP crystals showing a mass of numerous short rod-like crystals (× 10,400).

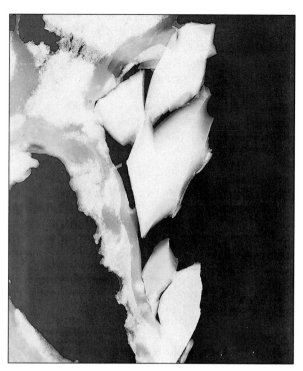

6.8 Electron micrograph of synovial fluid pellet showing plate-like crystals suggestive of octacalcium phosphate (× 22,200).

6.9

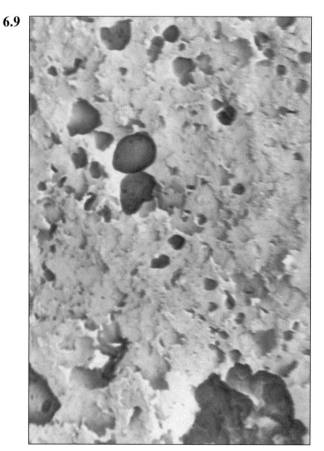

6.9 Scanning electron micrograph of a synovial fluid pellet showing microspheroids containing BCP crystals (× 1000).

Comment

What can be learned from the synovial fluid in OA? The factors which regulate synovial fluid accumulation in individual cases at any given time are largely unknown. Although referred to as 'non-inflammatory', the slightly elevated (compared to the completely normal joint) synovial leucocyte count probably reflects low-grade inflammation. This is also manifested in the osteoarthritic joint histology by patchy synovial lining cell hyperplasia (Doyle, 1982; Halverson *et al.*, 1984). The inflammatory stimulus is uncertain but may be related to cartilage fragments, crystals or other biochemical mediators. Severity of osteoarthritic articular symptoms has been associated with synovial leucocyte count and the presence of hydroxyapatite and other particulate matter (Schumacher, 1990).

BCP and CPPD crystals are frequently found in OA. In fact, they are found more commonly together than either is found alone (Gibilisco *et al.*, 1985; Halverson and McCarty, 1986). This has been referred to as 'mixed crystal deposition disease' (**6.10**) (Dieppe *et al.*, 1977). The significance of these two crystals occurring together is unknown. Although one could argue that joint degeneration associated with crystals does not constitute a pure form of OA, the entity called OA actually represents the final common pathway of a number of pathologic processes. The presence of BCP crystals has been correlated with more advanced radiographically apparent joint destruction than in

6.10

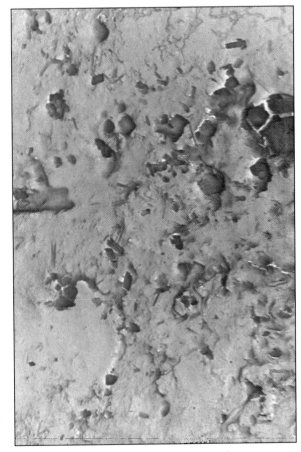

6.10 Scanning electron micrograph of a synovial fluid pellet showing microspheroids of BCP crystals and rhomboidal calcium pyrophosphate dihydrate crystals indicative of 'mixed crystal deposition' (× 1000).

OA without these crystals (Halverson and McCarty, 1979; Paul et al., 1983). CPPD crystal deposition has also been associated with OA-like changes but most reports have usually not included techniques that would have detected BCP crystals. One study found that CPPD crystal deposition appeared to be associated with age, whereas BCP crystal deposition was more associated with joint damage (Halverson and McCarty, 1986).

Although release of large amounts of crystals will cause an inflammatory attack of arthritis such as pseudogout or hydroxyapatite pseudopodagra (Fam and Rubenstein, 1989), low levels of crystals not exceeding some undefined threshold apparently do not generate a sufficient stimulus to recruit polymorphonuclear leucocytes to the joint space. This may be accounted for in part by the reduced ability of BCP crystals to generate cell movement factors from polymorphonuclear leucocytes on one hand and the increased surface binding of such factors by BCP on the other in comparison to monosodium urate monohydrate (Swan et al., 1990). Proteins adsorbed on to crystal surfaces probably modulate interactions with inflammatory cells. Terkeltaub et al. (1988) found that among the proteins found on BCP crystals, α_2-HS glycoprotein accounted for most of the inhibition of BCP-induced neutrophil superoxide release and chemiluminescence.

Experimental evidence has shown that collagen (Biswas and Dayer, 1979), hydroxyapatite and CPPD crystals (Cheung et al., 1981) elicit increased collagenase production and that cartilaginous wear particles elicit increased neutral protease production (Evans et al., 1981) in cell culture systems, but these phenomena have not been confirmed in vivo. Initial reports of 'Milwaukee shoulder syndrome', also called 'idiopathic destructive arthritis of the shoulder' (Campion et al., 1988) and 'cuff tear arthropathy' (Neer et al., 1983), described low levels of collagenase in some shoulder joint fluids in association with BCP crystals (Halverson et al., 1984). Other investigators have not found collagenase in synovial fluid from similar patients (Dieppe et al., 1988). Collagenase in low concentration may be difficult to detect because of its propensity to bind to collagen-containing tissue. It would seem difficult to explain the destruction of collagenous tissues without implicating collagenase in some way.

Interleukin-1 (IL-1) levels are low in synovial fluid from osteoarthritic joints in comparison with rheumatoid arthritis and other inflammatory arthropathies (Westacott et al., 1990). BCP crystals stimulate release of PGE_2 but not Il-1 from mouse macrophages (Alwan et al., 1988). Neutrophil activating peptide (Il-8) is demonstrable in the synovial fluid of patients with urate gout but not osteoarthritis (Terkeltaub et al., 1991). Thus, the cytokines Il-1 and Il-8 do not appear to be relevant to osteoarthritis. Tumour necrosis factor alpha (TNFα) was increased in osteoarthritis relative to rheumatoid arthritis (Westacott et al., 1990), but higher levels of TNFα were also found in two other non-inflammatory joint effusions not caused by osteoarthritis. Thus, in synovial fluid there appears to be surprising discordance between Il-1 and TNFa. Another enzyme that may have importance in generating inorganic pyrophosphate, nucleotide pyrophosphohydrolase, is increased in osteoarthritic synovial fluids but even more so in fluids containing BCP and CPPD crystals (Rachow et al., 1986).

In summary, osteoarthritic synovial fluid appears bland in comparison to more inflammatory conditions, yet BCP and CPPD crystals are often present. Whether these represent merely epiphenomena or contribute directly to joint destruction in osteoarthritis remains unknown. The roles of cytokines, prostaglandins, and possibly other factors and their affects cartilage chondrocytes, synoviocytes, and ultimately the process resulting in osteoarthritis have not yet been defined.

References and further reading

Alwan, W.H., Dieppe, P.A., Elson, C.J., Bradfield, J.W.B. (1988) Bone resorbing activity in synovial fluids in destructive osteoarthritis and rheumatoid arthritis. *Ann. Rheum. Dis.*, **47**, 198–205.

Bardin, T., Bucki, B., Lansaman, J., Ortiz Bravo, E., Ryckewaert, A., Dryll, A. (1987) Coloration par le rouge alizarine des liquides articulaires. *Rev. Rhum. Mal. Osteoartic.*, **54**, 149–154.

Biswas, C., Dayer, J. (1979) Stimulation of collagenase production by collagen in mammalian cell cultures. *Cell*, **18**, 1035–1041.

Blair, J.M., Ratneswar, L., Sorensen, L.B., Arnsdorf, M. (1992) Identification of hydroxyapatite and other synovial microcrystals by application of atomic force microscopy (AFM). *Arthritis Rheum.*, **35**, R27.

Campion, G.V., McCrae, F., Alwan, W., Watt, I., Bradfield, J., Dieppe, P.A. (1988) Idiopathic destructive arthritis of the shoulder. *Sem. Arthritis Rheum.*, **17**, 232–245.

Cherian, P.V., Schumacher, H.R. (1982) Diagnostic potential of rapid electron microscopy analysis of joint effusions. *Arthritis Rheum.*, **25**, 98–100.

Cheung, H.S., Halverson, P.B., McCarty, D.J. (1981) Release of collagenase, neutral protease, and prostaglandins from cultured mammalian synovial cells by hydroxyapatite and calcium pyrophosphate dihydrate crystals. *Arthritis Rheum.*, **24**, 1338–1344.

Dieppe, P.A., Cawston, T., Mercer, E., Campion, G.V., Hornby, J., Hutton, C.W., Doherty, M., Watt, I., Woolf, A.D., Hazleman, B. (1988) Synovial fluid collagenase in patients with destructive arthritis of the shoulder joint. *Arthritis Rheum.*, **31**, 882–890.

Dieppe, P.A., Crocker, P.R., Corke, C.F., Doyle, D.V., Huskisson, E.C., Willoughby, D.A. (1979) Synovial fluid crystals. *Quart. J. Med.*, **192**, 533–553.

Dieppe, P.A., Doherty, M., MacFarlane, D.G., Hutton, C.W. (1977) Mixed crystal deposition disease and osteoarthritis. *Br. Med. J.*, **1**, 150.

Doyle, D.V. (1982) Tissue calcification and inflammation in osteoarthritis. *J. Pathol.* **136**, 199–216.

Evans, C.H., Means, D.C., Cosgrove, J.R. (1981) Release of neutral proteinase from mononuclear phagocytes and synovial cells in response to cartilaginous wear particles in vitro. *Biochim. Biophys. Acta*, **677**, 287–294.

Fam, A.G., Rubenstein, J. (1989) Hydroxyapatite pseudopodagra. *Arthritis Rheum.*, **32**, 741–747.

Gibilisco, P.A., Schumacher, H.R., Hollander, J.L., Soper, K.A. (1985) Synovial fluid crystals in osteoarthritis. *Arthritis Rheum.*, **28**, 511–515.

Gordon, C., Swan, A., Dieppe, P. (1989) Detection of crystals in synovial fluids by light microscopy: sensitivity and reliability. *Ann. Rheum. Dis.*, **48**, 737–742.

Halverson, P.B., Garancis, J.C., McCarty, D.J. (1984) Histopathological and ultrastructural studies of synovium in Milwaukee shoulder syndrome – a basic calcium phosphate crystal arthropathy. *Ann. Rheum. Dis.*, **43**, 734–741.

Halverson, P.B., McCarty, D.J. (1979) Identification of hydroxyapatite crystals in synovial fluid. *Arthritis Rheum.*, **22**, 389–395.

Halverson, P.B., McCarty, D.J. (1986) Patterns of radiographic abnormalities associated with basic calcium phosphate and calcium pyrophosphate dihydrate crystal deposition in the knee. *Ann. Rheum. Dis.*, **45**, 603–605.

Halverson, P.B., McCarty, D.J., Cheung, H.S., Ryan, L.M. (1984) Milwaukee shoulder syndrome: eleven additional cases with involvement of the knee in seven. *Sem. Arthritis. Rheum.*, **14**, 36–44.

McCarty, D.J. (1993) Synovial fluid. In *Arthritis and Allied Conditions*. Lea & Febiger, London.

McCarty, D.J., Gatter, R.A. (1966) Recurrent acute inflammation associated with focal apatite crystal deposition. *Arthritis Rheum.*, **9**, 804–819.

McCarty, D.J., Lehr, J.R., Halverson, P.B. (1983) Crystal populations in human synovial fluid. Identification of apatite, octacalcium phosphate, and tricalcium phosphate. *Arthritis Rheum.*, **26**, 1220–1224.

Neer, C.S., Craig, E.V., Fukuda, H. (1983) Cuff tear arthropathy. *J. Bone Joint Surg.*, **69A**, 1232–1244.

Paul, H., Reginato, A.J., Schumacher, H.R. (1983) Alizarin red S staining as a screening test to detect calcium compounds in synovial fluid. *Arthritis Rheum.*, **26**, 191–200.

Rachow, J.W., Ryan, L.M., McCarty, D.J., Halverson, P.B. (1986) Synovial fluid inorganic pyrophosphate concentration and nucleotide pyrophosphohydrolase activity in basic calcium phosphate deposition arthropathy and Milwaukee shoulder syndrome. *Arthritis Rheum.*, **31**, 408–413.

Ropes, M.W., Bauer, W. (1953) In *Synovial fluid*. Harvard University Press, Cambridge.

Schumacher Jr., H.R., Stineman, M., Rahman, M., Magee, S., Huppert, A. (1990) The relationship between clinical and synovial fluid findings and treatment response in osteoarthritis (OA) of the knee. *Arthritis Rheum.*, **33**, S92.

Swan, A., Dularay, B., Dieppe, P. (1990) A comparison of the effects of urate, hydroxyapatite and diamond crystals on polymorphonuclear cells: relationship of mediator release to the surface area and adsorptive capacity of different particles. *J. Rheumatol.*, **17**, 1346–1352.

Terkeltaub, R., Zachariae, C., Santoro, D., Martin, J., Peveri, P., Matsushima, K. (1990) Il-8 as a potential mediator of crystal-induced synovitis. *Arthritis Rheum.*, **33**, S20.

Terkeltaub, R.A., Santoro, D.A., Mandel, G., Mandel, N. (1988) Serum and plasma inhibit neutrophil stimulation by hydroxyapatite crystals. *Arthritis Rheum.*, **31**, 1081–1088.

Westacott, C.I., Whicher, J.T., Barnes, I.C., Thompson, D., Swan, A.J., Dieppe, P.A. (1990) Synovial fluid concentrations of five different cytokines in rheumatic diseases. *Ann. Rheum. Dis.*, **49**, 676–681.

7. Endemic and Rare Metabolic Forms

Leon Sokoloff

Several inherently non-inflammatory deforming joint diseases resemble osteoarthritis (OA) to a varying degree. They are of diverse aetiology and pathogenesis and so are not readily classified into logically parallel categories. Emphasis is placed in this chapter on their pathology and pathogenesis. This is because, aside from intrinsic clinical significance, they may give insight into the pathogenesis of common varieties of OA. Three principal groups are distinguished here:

- Endemic.
- Hereditary pre-arthrotic.
- Metabolic.

Crystal deposition diseases are dealt with in other chapters.

Endemic OA

Two endemic forms of OA occur in remote parts of the world. They are distinct from the common varieties of OA in several ways. Both entities, Kashin–Beck disease and Mseleni disease, begin in pre-adolescent years, and affect growth plate as well as articular cartilage, causing diminished stature. Both diseases are of a severe, non-inflammatory, deforming nature, and involve multiple joints.

Kashin–Beck disease

This enigmatic disorder incapacitates about 2 million people in regions of north China (**7.1**). In some rural communities, the prevalence is 90% of the population. The Chinese name, *dagujiebing*, means big joint disease. The enlargement causes stiffness and pain. Osteochondritis dissecans supervenes and further deformity is self-procreating. Contractures of the joints and loose bodies are common. Finger joints are the earliest affected. The rays are shortened and the bony enlargement gives an impression of Heberden and Bouchard nodes (**7.2**). Other joints involved, in order of frequency, are: the wrists, ankles, knees, shoulders and hips. Established changes are irreversible. In early stages, removal of the child to a non-endemic location apparently leads to reversal of the changes or at least hinders the progression. In later stages, orthopaedic measures are used.

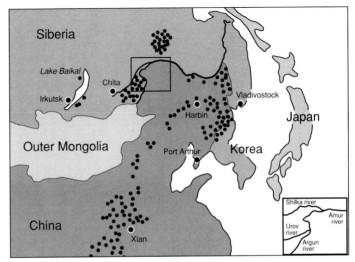

7.1

7.1 Geographical distribution of Kashin–Beck disease (with kind permission of *NY State J. Med.*).

The pathological anatomy of Kashin–Beck disease is unique: the earliest lesion is a zonal coagulation necrosis of the basal portion of the articular and growth plate cartilages (**7.3, 7.4**). Growth restriction is the consequence of premature union of the epiphyses (**7.5**). Osteophytic remodelling is responsible for enlargement of the joint (**7.6**). Environmental factors suggested as aetiological agents include selenium deficiency, and ingestion of mouldy grain or phenolic wood products among others. None has been proven (Li *et al.*, 1990; Sokoloff, 1989).

7.2

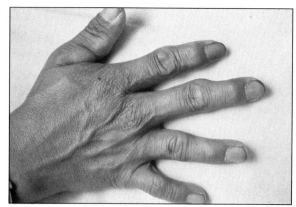

7.2 Characteristic finger deformities in Kashin–Beck disease. Enlarged interphalangeal joints resemble Heberden and Bouchard nodes. The rays are shortened (patient of Professor P.P. Yin). Reproduced with kind permission of *Clinics in Rheumatic Diseases*.

7.3

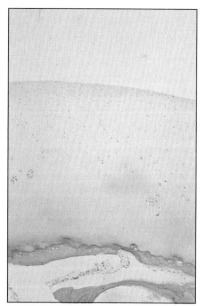

7.4

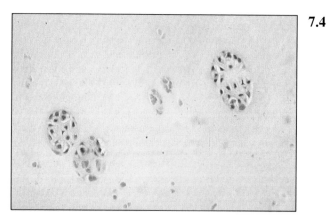

7.4 Higher magnification of **7.3**. Necrotic chondrocytes appear red rather than blue. Clones of chondrocytes have formed at the edge of the necrotic zone and within these clusters, individual cells have died. Thus the noxious process is ongoing or episodic.

7.3 Chondronecrosis of articular cartilage in early Kashin–Beck disease. Pallor of the basal field reflects the zonal character of the necrosis (case of Professor D.X. Mo). Reproduced with kind permission of *Clinics in Rheumatic Diseases*.

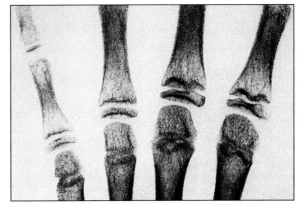

7.5 Radiograph of hand in early Kashin–Beck disease. Premature and uneven ossification of the growth plate is seen in the second and third metacarpal heads.

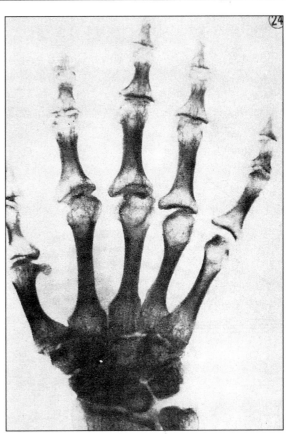

7.6 Advanced radiological changes in Kashin–Beck disease. The joint surfaces are broadened, spaces narrowed, rays shortened and variably subluxated.

Mseleni joint disease

Approximately 3,000 people living in the vicinity of the village of Mseleni in Northern Zululand are affected by a crippling, polyarticular non-inflammatory joint disease. At one time, 42% of the women in the area and 19% of men were affected. The condition manifests itself during the first decade of life. The hip joint is consistently involved, followed in order by the ankle, knee, wrist, shoulder and elbow. The fully developed radiological changes in the hip are those of severe coxarthrosis (**7.7**) or protrusio acetabuli, but in the adolescent the femoral head has a rather jagged pattern of ossification. The pathological changes in surgically resected hips (Sokoloff *et al.*,

1985) are much like those found in some instances of the precocious osteoarthritis associated with multiple epiphyseal dysplasias discussed later in this chapter (**7.8, 7.9**). Thus in its pathology, predilection for the hip and demographic considerations, Mseleni disease bears little similarity to Kashin–Beck disease. Some believe (Solomon *et al.*, 1986) that we are not dealing with a single entity. Rather, most of the disorder is an hereditary epiphyseal dysplasia. This runs contrary to genetic analyses conducted by others. If Mseleni disease is of environmental origin, the causative factor is entirely unknown.

7.7

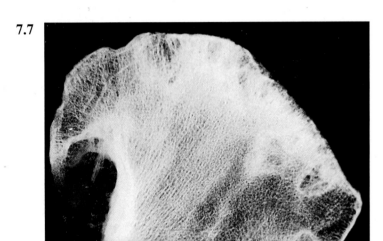

7.7 Radiograph of coronal slab section of femoral head in Mseleni hip disease. The changes resemble those of conventional coxarthrosis. Reproduced with kind permission of *Human Pathology*.

7.

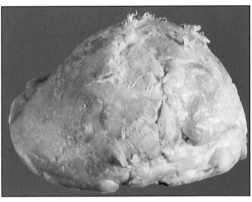

7.8 Deformity of femoral head in Mseleni disease, frontal view. The entire cartilage appears shaggy but there is no eburnation. A shelf-like osteophyte protrudes from the lateral margin on the left. Reproduced with kind permission of *Human Pathology*.

7.9

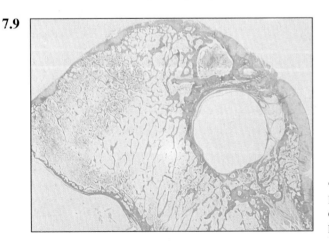

7.9 Photomicrograph of femoral head in Mseleni disease. A large subchondral pseudocyst is present, but a tattered cartilage covers the articular surface. Reproduced with kind permission of *Human Pathology*.

Hereditary pre-arthrotic disorders

Certain inherited abnormalities of articular cartilage and of bone lead to precocious degenerative joint disease. The pathogenic mechanisms of the destruction of cartilage are quite different in the two tissue categories.

Multiple epiphyseal and spondylo-epiphyseal dysplasias

These heterogeneous chondrodystrophies have varying inheritance patterns, sites of predilection and sometimes identifiably different cellular abnormalities. Several chromosomal and allelic mutants of type II procollagen have recently been identified (Ala-Kokka et al., 1990; Tiller et al., 1990). Spondylo-epiphyseal dysplasias have, in addition to the appendicular joint features, platyspondyly (7.10, 7.11). In certain forms, the dysplasia is confined to one joint, typically the hip (Learmonth et al., 1987). The process is, so far as can be determined from radiographic examination, characterised by delayed and irregular ossification as well as fragmentation of the epiphysis and growth plate. The articular ends are deformed thereby, commonly with disproportionate dwarfism. Precocious OA supervenes, particularly in the hip (Stanescu et al., 1987). In surgically resected specimens, the contour is abnormal apart from osteophytic remodelling (7.12). The articular cartilage is tattered, thinned and fibrotic. Subchondral sclerosis and pseudocysts are seen in the radiographs but eburnation is often absent. The pathological process thus has certain similarities to ordinary OA but there are also differences. Although abnormalities of the chondrocytes underlie the dysplasia, one can only speculate about the relative contributions of their abnormal metabolic products versus the disturbed mechanical loading resulting from the deformity.

7.10

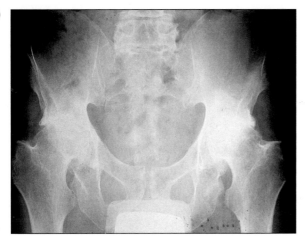

7.10 Hip joints of a 33-year-old man with spondylo-epiphyseal dysplasia. The radiographic appearance is that of predominantly superior pole OA (patient of Dr M. Doherty).

7.11

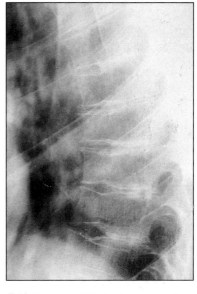

7.11 Platyspondyly in the same patient as shown in **7.10**. Anteroposterior elongation of the vertebral bodies, and marked intervertebral narrowing with 'fish mouth' abnormality in the anterior portions are characteristic.

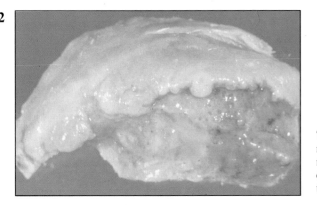

7.12 Femoral head resected from a 47-year-old woman with multiple epiphyseal dysplasia. The head is flattened and marginal osteophytes are covered by white cartilage. The cartilage is thinned and eburnation is present over much of the surface.

Osteopetrosis

Most people who have hereditary osteopetrosis die young from the myelophthisic complications. The genetic defect leaves chondroclasts unable to remove calcified cartilage (7.13) or osteoclasts to remove membranous bone from the primary skeletal template. Thus there is no marrow space for haematopoietic tissue. The bulk of the 'marble bone' actually consists of calcified cartilage (7.14). Although the bone is very hard, it fractures frequently, apparently breaking because of stress concentration along the osteochondral planes (7.15). Remodelling sequences are also interrupted and the shape of the bone is deformed through deficient metaphyseal cutback. The weight of the bones itself imposes a mechanical burden in locomotion.

In the small proportion of individuals who survive into the fifth decade of life, degenerative joint disease occurs (7.16) (Milgram and Jasty, 1982). Total joint replacements have been reported (Casden *et al.*, 1988). The occurrence of OA in osteopetrosis has been cited as evidence in support of a theory that stiffness of underlying bone is the principal mechanical basis for cartilage degeneration in ordinary OA. The association with fractures here, however, makes this interpretation overly simple.

7.13

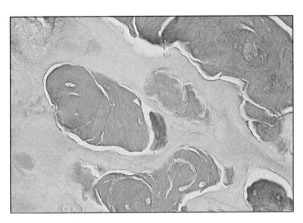

7.13 Photomicrograph of osteopetrosis. The blue-stained material is cartilage; the red, woven bone. Absence of nuclei indicates that the long-standing mineralisation of these matrices has caused the cells to die.

7.14

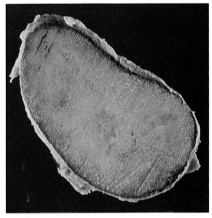

7.14 Marble bone appearance of cross-section of femoral shaft in osteopetrosis. There is no medullary cavity.

7.15

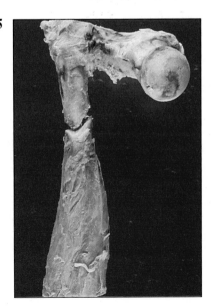

7.15 Two fractures are seen in the femoral diaphysis: one, in the subtro-chanteric region, is old and united in a markedly angulated deformity. The more distal discontinuity is a post-mortem artefact resulting from the brittleness of the bone. The bulbous enlargement of the shaft exemplifies the faulty metaphyseal cutback process.

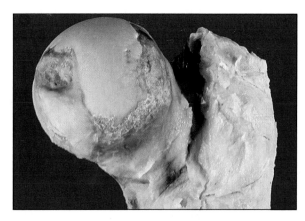

7.16 Atrophy and fibrillation of articular cartilage of femoral head in same specimen as in **7.15**. The patient was 31 years old and had been bedridden for years. Mechanical wear was thus not a tenable mechanism for these osteoarthritic changes.

Metabolic arthropathies

Forms of osteoarthritis that have their inception in articular cartilage may usefully be called chondrogenic to distinguish them from those that arise from mechanical disturbances. The damaging agents may be hormones or toxic metals or organic compounds. They may have analogies in clinical evidence that certain non-steroidal anti-inflammatory drugs (Rashad *et al.*, 1989) and chemotherapeutic agents (Martel-Pelletier, 1986) may potentiate development of ordinary OA.

Haemochromatosis

The iron overload disorder, haemochromatosis, comes about through two different pathways:

- A primary or idiopathic one in which iron accumulates through some genetically determined abnormality of the turnover mechanism of the metal.
- A secondary variety in which there is a massive overloading by breakdown of large amounts of haemoglobin, e.g. in the thalassaemias.

Often the condition is not recognised until late in life, or even until after death. The classic complications of cellular iron storage occur in liver, pancreas and myocardium, but joints, too, are commonly affected. A recent survey by the Hemochromatosis Research Foundation in the USA indicated that arthropathy was the most common feature of the idiopathic form (Schumacher, 1988).

Most joints can be affected but osteoarthritic changes of the metacarpophalangeals and wrist are most typical (**7.17**). In this the distribution is rather like that of chondrocalcinosis. Indeed, calcium pyro-phosphate dihydrate crystal deposition occurs in approximately one-third of cases. The presumptive mechanism is inhibition of inorganic pyrophosphatase by the Fe(III). There are few reports of the morbid anatomy of the arthropathy. A consistent finding is a fine stippling of synovial lining cells with Fe(III) (**7.18**). In articular cartilage, too, iron has been found within the cytoplasm of chondrocytes (Schumacher, 1988) but not in the matrix. Iron must necessarily have traversed the matrix to reach the cell. The latter presumably serves as a sink to keep the cation from harming the matrix.

The radiological finding of osteopenia in haemochromatosis results from an iron osteopathy. Iron is deposited along cement lines and the endosteal surface in thalassaemias (Laeng *et al.*, 1988) (**7.19**). Subsequent development of osteomalacia suggests a mechanism analogous to that of aluminium osteopathy: the trivalent cation at the mineralising front interferes with the deposition of hydroxyapatite in the adjacent osteoid seam.

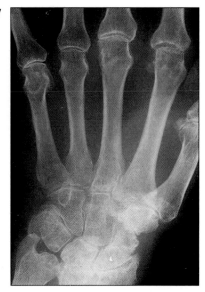

7.17 Radiographic appearance of haemochromatotic arthropathy in a 47-year-old patient. There is an eccentric loss of metacarpophalangeal and radiocarpal joint spaces. A hook osteophyte is present on the fifth metacarpal head. The distribution together with absence of scaphoid-lunate dissociation is quite characteristic of this disease. (Patient of Dr M. Doherty.)

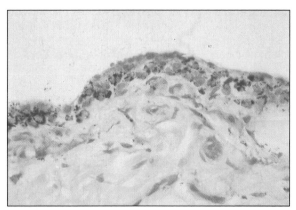

7.18 Iron stored in synovial lining cells in haemochromatosis is manifested by fine Prussian blue-stained material. (Perls' stain.)

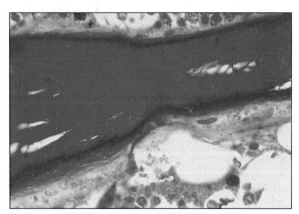

7.19 Iron osteopathy in haemochromatosis. Prussian blue-stained material is present along the endosteal surface but none was seen in articular chondrocytes in this case.

Haemophilic arthropathy

Recurrent haemarthrosis occurs in approximately 90% of those afflicted with major haemophilias. Acute episodes are painful but over the long term lead to permanent destructive changes in the joints. Often there is an intermediate stage that resembles OA radiologically and pathologically (7.20, 7.21). Just how the extravasation of blood causes joint destruction is uncertain; multiple mechanisms are probably involved (Madhok *et al.*, 1988). Resorption of the blood by synovial lining cells and macrophages leads to marked haemosiderosis of the capsular tissues (7.22). Articular cartilage apparently disappears rapidly, but in residual tissue, chondrocytes contain stainable Fe(III). None is seen in the matrix. There are two possibilities by which the Fe(III) may damage cartilage:

- As in haemochromatosis, the cation in passage may interact with the sulfated proteoglycans of the matrix electrostatically, thereby causing loss of elasticity and rapid mechanical abrasion.
- The iron overload may exceed the iron-binding capacity of the synovial fluid, so that ionic ('free') iron can react with the articular tissues.

There is some evidence for both possibilities. The iron is capable of participating in oxygen-free radical formation. Another possibility is that enzymes released from damaged cells during the erythrophagocytosis may act on the tissues. Autoimmune reactions have also been suggested but immunocytic infiltration is not ordinarily seen in the lesions. Intramedullary haemorrhage is also present and causes pseudocyst formation. Elevated intra-articular pressure and immobilisation may well contribute to the deformities.

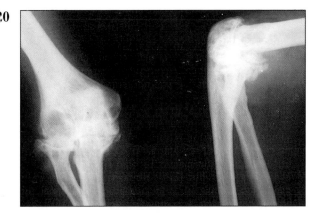

7.20 Osteoarthritic phase of haemophilic arthropathy of the elbow. The joint space is narrowed and osteophytic spurs protrude from the margins of the olecranon and distal humerus (patient of Dr M. Gilbert).

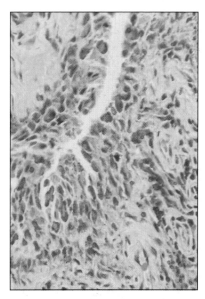

7.22 Synovium in haemophilic arthropathy. Large amounts of coarse golden granules of haemosiderin are present in the cytoplasm of lining cells and deeper macrophages.

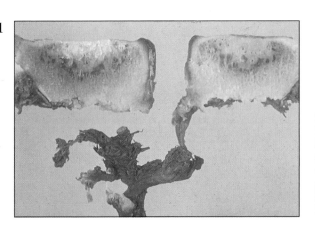

7.21 Radial head resected from the same patient as in **7.20**. The attached synovial tissue is thickened and rust-coloured. Cartilage has disappeared from most of the humeral articulating surface but some persists on the ulnar aspect. A wedge-shaped area of subchondral sclerosis and pigmentation is present beneath the abraded surface. Reproduced with kind permission of *Archives of Pathology*, 1976, **100**, 91–96. © 1976 American Medical Association.

Wilson's disease

Wilson's disease, a rare hereditary defect of copper metabolism, leads to accumulation of toxic quantities of copper in many organs and so to cirrhosis of the liver, lenticular degeneration with movement disorders, and Keyser–Fleischer rings of the cornea. The large majority of patients have joint complaints – mostly in the knee, but also in other diarthroses and the lumbosacral spine as well. The clinical features are those of a precocious generalised degenerative joint disease but there is little morphological documentation of the state of the joints. Although often referred to as an OA, the radiological features are atypical (Resnick and Niwayama, 1988). The joint space is narrowed but the subchondral plate appears irregular rather than eburnated. Osteopenia is present – whether it is simply osteoporotic or osteomalacic is not known. The pathogenesis is uncertain. No correlation has been established with the severity of the neurological impairment and a neuropathic basis is not supported thereby. Calcium pyrophosphate dihydrate crystal deposition, theoretically possible through inhibition of inorganic pyrophosphatase by Cu(II), is not commonly found. There is some evidence that copper levels in articular tissues are elevated (Menerey et al., 1988).

Ochronosis

Ochronosis is relatively rare but commands recognition as a possible prototype of systemic factors that contribute to what now appear to be primary forms of generalised OA. Here the aetiological factor is recognised through its colour marker, while colourless contributors would be less easily recognised.

Most instances of ochronosis are of hereditary nature and result from a defective homogentisic acid oxidase. Homogentisic acid (HGA), a partial degradation product of tyrosine and phenylalanine, is excreted into the urine. In the presence of oxygen, urinary HGA is converted into a melanin-like pigment – hence the term alkaptonuria. Formation of ochronotic pigment within the body does not occur as rapidly. The author has seen costal cartilage from one 10-year-old patient in which there was no discolouration. Extrinsic phenolic compounds have historically been known to cause instances of ochronosis. At present, the only chemicals known to cause ochronotic pigmentation are topical hydroquinone-containing cosmetics. Here the ochronosis is confined to the immediate cutaneous tissues. It is, perhaps, surprising that L-dopa and dopaminergic medications commonly used to treat parkinsonism do not produce ochronosis. A rare instance has been seen, but so too has spontaneous association of the two entities reported in an individual not so treated (Siekert and Gibilisco, 1970). Perhaps the duration of such medication is insufficient for ochronosis to develop. Despite the obtrusiveness of pigmentation, there are instances of ochronosis in which the condition is first recognised at surgery or necropsy.

The hyaline cartilages and intervertebral discs are the sites of pigment deposition. A feature of articular pigmentation is a predilection for the radial zone. Other connective tissues (heart valves, sclerae, renal pyramids and dermis) are also pigmented to varying degree, but bone is spared. The pigmented tissues undergo necrobiosis and become brittle. Loss of mechanical strength leads to disintegration of the cartilages and thereby to generalised OA. Shards of detached cartilage provoke secondary osteochondromatous metaplasia of the synovium (**7.23, 7.24**) that may appear as loose bodies in radiographs.

Axial as well as appendicular joints are affected. Pigmentation of intervertebral discs is followed in time by mineralisation. Most of this is an ossific process (Gaines, 1989) but calcification alone is often described without clear documentation. In about 20% of cases, acute disc displacement is the presenting complaint; but spondylosis, often with ankylosis, kyphosis and loss of height, is the end result.

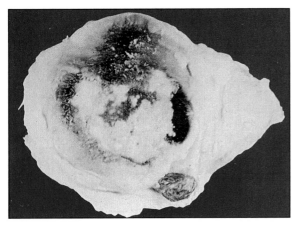

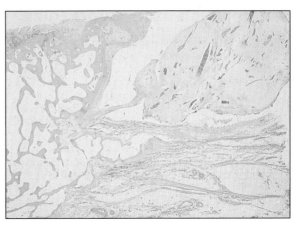

7.23 Ochronosis of patella. The surface has areas of fibrillation, exposure of ebony black cartilage and denuded foci of non-pigmented eburnated bone. The polypoid structure at the lower right is a secondary osteochondromatous reaction to shards of cartilage displaced into the synovium. Reproduced with kind permission of *Arthritis Rheumatism*.

7.24 Photomicrograph from the same specimen as in **7.23**. Pigmented fragments of cartilage in the polyp reflect the brittle nature of the ochronotic cartilage. Reproduced with kind permission of *Arthritis Rheumatism*.

Acromegaly

Approximately three out of four acromegalic patients complain of pain in their finger joints or in large peripheral joints. Early on, this is the consequence of hypertrophy of articular cartilage and adjacent connective tissues, detectable in radiographs, but proceeds to secondary degenerative changes that closely resemble generalised OA (**7.25**). Periosteal membranous new bone formation is the counterpart in the vertebral column and facial bones. The pathological findings in patients who have undergone total hip replacement are almost identical to those of ordinary OA (Johanson, 1985). One pathological feature, however, carries a more generalised significance for OA: a moderate chronic synovitis is present in most. This is prima facie evidence that the capsular inflammation, commonly present in surgical OA, is indeed a secondary phenomenon.

The cartilaginous and periosteal hypertrophy result from the action of somatotropin (growth hormone, GH) released by eosinophilic pituitary adenomas. For many years, it has been taught that GH does not act directly on the chondrocytes but rather a GH-dependent liver product, insulin-like growth factor 1. There is, however, some evidence that at least certain chondrocytes may be direct targets of GH (Werther *et*

al., 1990). Age may determine the susceptibility to the two hormones. In any event, once the hypertrophic changes have developed, treatment by surgical extirpation, irradiation or administration of somatostatin analogues does little or nothing to halt the arthropathy (Dons *et al.*, 1988; Layton *et al.*, 1988). For this reason caution has been recommended in treating real or perceived shortness of stature with recombinant GH. The findings are also relevant to some experimental evidence that an early response to mechanical instability of a joint may be hypertrophy of articular cartilage, and that osteoarthritic changes develop slowly thereafter (Adams, 1989).

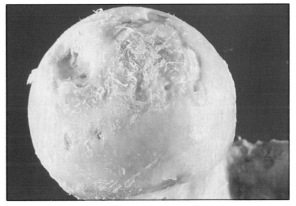

7.25 Acromegalic arthropathy of hip joint. The patient was a 40-year-old woman whose pituitary gland had been extirpated for an eosinophilic adenoma at the age of 10 years. There is an area of deep fibrillation of the cartilage on the posterior aspect of the femoral head. A pointed osteophyte was present anteriorly.

References and further reading

Adams, M.E. (1989) Cartilage hypertrophy following canine anterior cruciate ligament transection differs among different areas of the joint. *J. Rheumatol.*, **16**, 818–824.

Ala-Kokka, L., Baldwin, C.T., Moskowitz, R.W., Prockop, D.J. (1990) Single base mutation in the type II procollagen gene (COL2A1) as a cause of primary osteoarthritis associated with mild chondrodysplasia. *Proc. Natl. Acad. Sci. USA*, **87**, 6565–6568.

Casden, A.M., Jaffe, F.F., Kastenbaum, D.M., Bonar, S.F. (1988) Osteoarthritis associated with osteopetrosis treated by total knee arthroplasty. *Clin. Orth. Rel. Res.*, **247**, 202–207.

Dons, R.F., Rosselet, P., Pastakia, B., Doppman, J., Gorden, P. (1988) Arthropathy in acromegalic patients before and after treatment. *Clin. Endocrinol.*, **28**, 515–524.

Gaines, J.J., Jr. (1989) The pathology of alkaptonuric ochronosis. *Hum. Pathol.*, **20**, 40–46.

Johanson, N.A. (1985) Endocrine arthropathies. *Clin. Rheum. Dis.*, **11**, 297–323.

Laeng, H., Egger, T., Roethlisberger, C., Cottier, H. (1988) Stainable bone iron in undecalcified, plastic-embedded sections. Occurrence in man related to the presence of 'free' iron? *Am. J. Pathol.*, **131**, 344–350.

Layton, M.W., Fudman, E.J., Barkan, A., Braunstein, E.M., Fox, I.H. (1988) Acromegalic arthropathy. Characteristics and response to therapy. *Arth. Rheum.*, **31**, 1022–1027.

Learmonth, I.D., Christy, G., Beighton, P. (1987) Namaqualand hip dysplasia: orthopedic implications. *Clin. Orthop. Rel. Res.*, **218**, 142–147.

Li, F.S., Duan, Y.J., Yan, S.J., *et al.* (1990) Presenile (early ageing) changes in tissue in Kashin–Beck disease and its pathogenic significance. *Mech. Ageing Dev.*, **54**, 103–120.

Madhok, R., Bennett, D., Sturrock, R.D., Forbes, C.D. (1988) Mechanisms of joint damage in an experimental model of haemophilic arthritis. *Arth. Rheum.*, **31**, 1148–1155.

Martel-Pelletier, J., Pelletier, J.P. (1986) Degradative changes in human articular cartilage induced by chemotherapeutic agents. *J. Rheumatol.*, **13**, 164–174.

Menerey, K.A., Eider, W., Brewer, G.J., Braunstein, E.M., Schumacher, R., Fox, I.H. (1988) The arthropathy of Wilson's disease: clinical and pathological features. *J. Rheumatol.*, **15**, 331–337.

Milgram, J.W., Jasty, M. (1982) Osteopetrosis: a morphological study of twenty-one cases. *J. Bone Joint Surg.*, **64A**, 912–929.

Rashad, S., Revell, P., Hemingway, A., Low, F., Rainsford, K., Walker, F. (1989) Effect of non-steroidal anti-inflammatory drugs on the course of osteoarthritis. *Lancet*, **2**, 519–521.

Resnick, D., Niwayama, G. (1988) *'Diagnosis of Bone and Joint Disorders.* 2nd ed. Vol. 3, 1779–1786. W.B. Saunders, Philadelphia.

Schumacher, H.R., Straka, P.C., Krikker, M.A., Dudley, A.T. (1988) The arthropathy of hemochromatosis. Recent studies. *Ann. N.Y. Acad. Sci.*, **526**, 224–233.

Siekert, R.G., Gibilisco, J.A. (1970) Discoloration of the teeth in alkaptonuria (ochronosis) and parkinsonism. *Oral Surg., Oral Med., Oral Pathol.*, **29**, 197–199.

Sokoloff, L. (1989) The history of Kashin–Beck disease. *N.Y. State J. Med.*, **89**, 343–351.

Sokoloff, L., Fincham, J.E., du Toit, G.T. (1985) Pathologic features of the femoral head in Mseleni disease. *Hum. Pathol.*, **16**, 117–120.

Solomon, L., McLaren, P., Irwig, L., Gear, J.S.S., *et al.* (1986) Distinct types of hip disorder in Mseleni joint disease. *S.A. J. Med. Sci.*, **69**, 15–17.

Stanescu, R., Stanescu, V., Bordat, C., Maroteaux, P. (1987) Pathologic features of the femoral heads in a patient $14\frac{1}{2}$ years old with spondylo-epiphyseal dysplasia with osteoarthritis. *J. Rheumatol.*, **14**, 1061–1067.

Tiller, G.E., Rimoin, D.L., Murray, L.W., Cohn, D.H. (1990) Tandem duplication within a type II collagen gene (COL2A1) exon in an individual with spondylo-epiphyseal dysplasia. *Proc. Natl. Acad. Sci. USA*, **87**, 3889–3893.

Werther, G.A., Haynes, K.M., Barnard, R., Waters, M.J. (1990) Visual demonstration of growth hormone receptors on human growth plate chondrocytes. *J. Clin. Endocrinol. Metabol.*, **70**, 1725–1731.

8. Evolutionary Aspects of Osteoarthritis

Charles Hutton

Features of osteoarthritis (OA) have been described across the animal phylogenetic spectrum – in birds, reptiles and mammals. Detailed analysis is not available and there is always a danger of inconsistency in reporting features. However, the features of osteophyte formation are widespread so the osteoarthritic process of similar processes occur widely. Analysis is difficult because in the wild the predator competition means that any disability makes animals vulnerable, and remains are quickly destroyed by scavengers. Captivity avoids this but subjects the animal to an artificial environment. Nevertheless, the demonstration of OA in any example of a disparate species to man shows its potential ubiquity in the natural world. If it is ubiquitous, so too must be the underlying mechanisms. Insight into this common mechanism comes from evolutionary perspective and awareness of comparative zoology of joints.

The features of OA are first reviewed. Cartilage degeneration with fibrillation and crater formation occurs in a patchy distribution in the joint. There is an anabolic response with capsule fibrosis, subchondral sclerosis and osteophyte formation. With the osteophyte formation is the proliferation of new blood vessels, new cartilage with characteristics of immature cartilage rather than senescent cartilage. There may be duplication of the tide mark. These features have a parallel with the mechanisms of growth needed to produce a joint. Moreover, the natural experiments of the development of a pseudarthrosis following failed fracture healing, and the growth of cartilage in acromegaly indicates that the potential for new growth is latent in joints after skeletal maturation. Finally, in man, there is a distinctive temporal and special pattern of joint involvement. Joints developing disease early and commonly, such as the first metatarsal joint, contrast with those that develop it rarely and late, such as the ankle.

Comparative zoology undermines the simplistic approach to a 'wear and tear' ageing phenomenon. Some animals, particularly reptiles, live for up to a century, and no extraordinarily high incidence of joint disease is recognised in them. Animals vary considerably in their biological age. Man is unique in having a long immature period and a menopausal phase in the female stopping reproduction before the lifecycle ends. Man is also a cultural animal using tools.

The concept of OA as a final common pathway of joint failure means universality would be expected. Animals have a genetic constraint on the range of options they can produce, so a joint must have limits in the way it can respond to insult. To clarify: the animal's genome contains enough information to produce a new animal and to allow it to function. The amount of information is limited – by how much is unclear, but it does not contain information to produce just anything; the important feature is the limitation. It must contain some system coding the information needed to allow a joint to form. This system will be constrained by a dilemma of ensuring accurate transmission of information but being transferable. Space is limited. The system therefore must represent a compromise, which has two consequences:

- First, only information with a selection advantage needs to be transmitted. Most important is the system to develop a new animal – to make a joint and control its growth. A system to counter the effect of malfunction is less important, and in order to contain information transfer there is potential advantage in using systems for development in repair.
- Second, the system for joint maintenance may break down and trigger an osteoarthritic process, just as injury will trigger a mechanism for repair, which seems very similar to the initial process of joint growth. The design of the animal can be seen as an interaction between form and function generated by natural selection at several levels, information transfer and joint action being examples. Failure can then be intrinsic to the system as well as extrinsically produced by the environment.

Emergence and evolution of joints

It is necessary to consider the evolution of joints and human evolution (**8.1**). Joints are first seen in the Ordovician fish over 500 million years ago. They evolve with the emergence of amphibians 395 million years ago in the form of an appendicular skeletal allowing quadrupedal locomotion. This basic pattern is then modified into bipedal locomotion and flight by the diversification of reptiles during the Carboniferous period (345 million years ago). Mammals emerge during the Cretaceous period (110 million years ago). As a parallel step in the evolution of joints mammals, some birds and a few reptiles developed epiphyseal growth. Moreover in birds and mammals the epiphysis closes to stop growth. In contrast, animals such as crocodiles can continue to grow throughout life. Their growth slows with age but it does not stop.

Man emerges during the Pleistocene period with evidence of modern man, *Homo sapiens sapiens*, emerging less than a million years ago (**8.2**). The earliest evidence of bipedalism is 3.5 million years old with foot prints of a small bipedal hominid preserved at Laetoli in Tanzania (**8.3**). The ancestral lineage is controversial. However, contemporaneous with the Laetoli foot prints was a hominid, *Australopithecus afarensis*, that was bipedal (**8.4–8.6**). Near-complete skeletal material is available on specimens from the Hadar depression in Ethiopia. The most celebrated specimen is 'Lucy'. She shows features suggestive of partial adaptation, such as round rather than flattened femoral condyles and a larger lateral condyle, as well as laterally orientated acetabulae.

8.1

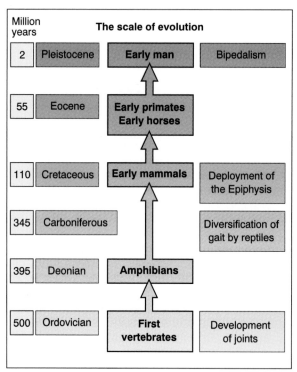

8.1 Scale of evolution.

8.

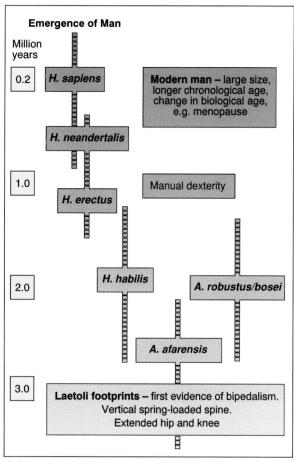

8.2 Emergence of man.

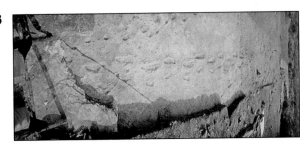

8.3 Laetoli foot prints (from Napier, J.R., Napier, P.H. *The natural history of the primates*, p.180).

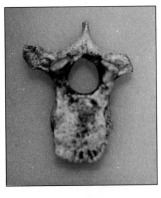

8.4 Spinal osteophytosis in *A. afarensis* (from a cast in the British Museum of Natural History).

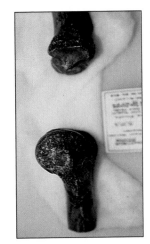

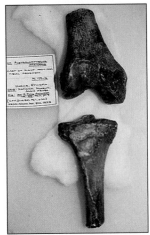

8.5, 8.6 Transitional features of the knee of *A. afarensis* (from a cast in the British Museum of Natural History).

Around 2 million years ago the first *homo* emerges, *Homo habilis*, still about half the height of modern man. This was superceded by *Homo erectus* (around 1.5 million years ago) who shows much more similar skeletal morphology to archaic *Homo sapiens* and was taller. *H. sapiens* begins to be seen about 0.5 million years ago. The lineage is unclear as until 0.2 million years ago a possible subspecies, *H. sapiens neandertalis*, was found in Eurasia. These were more robust than modern man and it is unclear whether they were an evolutionary off-shoot or an ancestor of modern man.

This lineage means that the modern skeletal morphology has only recently been established. That morphology reflects adaptation to bipedalism from some form of quadrupedal gait that was being established 3.5 million years ago. The changes are therefore recent and the equation of form to function may not be stabilised. Moreover, very recently there have been big changes in chronological and biological age. There is no evidence to suggest longevity was a common feature until very recently, and it has become widespread only in the past century with industrialisation. *H. neandertalis* probably only lived to 40 years. In contrast to other mammals, women have a menopausal stop to their reproductive period with the potential to post-reproductive life and a period when selection pressures on the genome will be indirect. Finally, over the past 2 million years there has been the development of tool use.

Man, then, has emerged recently with a rapid transformation of skeletal morphology, has increased in size, increased his longevity and changed biological lifecycle as well as developing culture.

This lineage is based on fossil evidence. In addition to allowing morphological change to be traced, these fossils also show that the early hominids had features of OA (**8.7, 8.8**). Lucy has degenerative change in her spine and evidence of spinal osteophytosis. The post-cranial remains from Kabwe in Zambia, which are possibly transitional from *H. erectus* to *H. sapiens*, in the hip. Most dramatically, Neanderthal man from La Chapelleaux-Saints shows extensive spinal apophyseal joint OA and evidence of Schmorl's nodes.

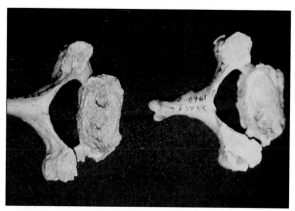

8.7 Rim osteophyte in *H. rhodesiensis* (from a cast in the British Museum of Natural History).

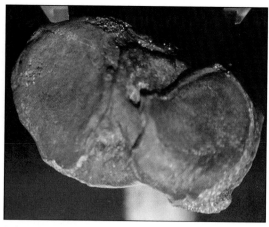

8.8 Apophyseal OA in *H. neandertalis* (Musée de L'Homme, Paris).

8.9

Million years	Emergence of the horse	
0	North America	Europe
	Extinction	
	Equus	One-toed manus and pes
10		Hipparon
15	Adaptive radiation	
	Central digit dominance. Increased body size. ?Increased longevity	
25	Parahippus	
35	Orohippus	
45	Hyracotherium	30kg Manus 4 digits, pes 3 digits. Plantigrade posture

8.9 Evolution of the horse.

Evolution of the horse

A comparable evolutionary perspective can be seen in the horse (**8.9**). This emerges as a small forest-dweller walking plantigrade 45 million years ago to become digitagrade and undergo an adaptive radiation about 15 million years ago from which the modern equus developed as a larger one-toed digitagrade animal (**8.10**). This emerged in the New World but survived only in Eurasia. More recently, it has been subjected to artificial selection and use after domestication by man. The pattern of osteoarthritic change in the horse skeleton reflects the joints showing this change in locomotion (**8.11**). In particular, it is rare in the hip and knee, and common in the foot itself, particularly the fetlock joint (**8.12, 8.13**).

In the horse, as in man, the features of osteophytosis associated with cartilage disintegration are comparable. This occurs most often in joints that have undergone recent morphological and functional change. That change has been powered by natural selection from an ancestral quadrupedal gait. Joints taking increased load patterns will then be functioning near their 'design' limit. This contrasts with joints that are less loaded and have then a high functional reserve, with a consequent low rate of failure (**8.14**).

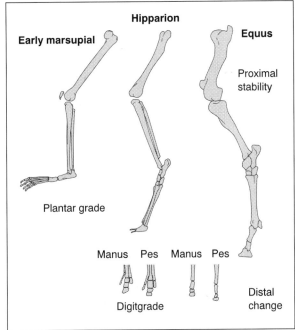

8.10 Change in limb configuration in horse evolution.

8.11 Pattern of OA in the horse.

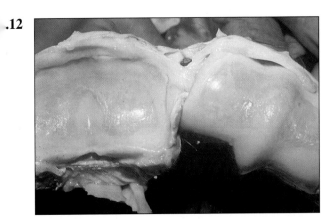

8.12 OA of the fetlock joint in the horse (courtesy of Dr Armstrong, Exeter University).

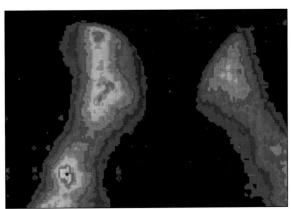

8.13 Bone scan of OA of the fetlock joint in the horse (courtesy of Dr W. Vennart, Exeter University).

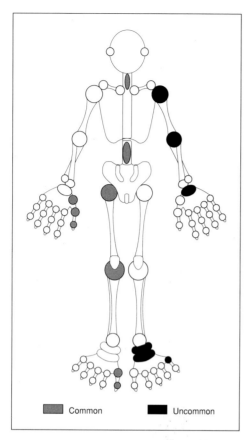

8.14 Distribution of OA in man.

Summary

The evolutionary perspective then allows:

- Recognition that the process of OA is a distinct biological response.
- Recognition that the distribution of OA in the skeleton may reflect the distribution of joints that are likely to be relatively underdesigned.
- Recognition that the failure of joints with age in primary OA may be caused by intrinsic breakdown of the systems controlling joint remodelling and maintenance.

References

Hutton, C.W. (1987) Generalised osteoarthritis, an evolutionary problem? *Lancet*, **i**, 1436–1465.
Hamerman, D. (1989) The biology of osteoarthritis. *N. Engl. J. Med.*, **320**, 1322–1330.
Radin, E.L., Paul, I.L., Rose, R.M. (1989) Osteoarthritis as the final common pathway. In *Aetiopathogenesis of osteoarthritis*, Nuki, G. (Ed.), Pitman Medical, 1979.

Suggested reading

Day, M.H. (1986) *Guide to fossil man*. Cassell, London.

9. Medical Management

Michael Shipley

General approach to the patient

The clinical manifestations of OA are extremely variable. Asymptomatic radiological changes are common and in an older patient should be noted, but no further action taken – the older the patient, the greater the likelihood of OA changes on X-rays. By 70 years of age nearly 100% have some evidence of radiological OA. In a significant number of patients the radiological appearances, especially if minor, are coincidental to any symptoms and merely reflect their age. **Local soft tissue causes of pain**, proximal origins of referred pain or the possibility of a more generalised pain syndrome such as **fibromyalgia** (see below) must all be considered before deciding the diagnosis is symptomatic OA. The key to correct management is a careful locomotor examination to establish an accurate diagnosis. This presumes a good knowledge of peri-articular structures and their potential for causing painful but often remediable problems. The medical approaches to OA are summarised in **Table 9.1**.

There is an inexplicably wide variation of symptoms between individuals who appear to have similar degrees of radiological abnormality. One may be virtually chair-bound by hip or knee involvement, while another, with similar appearances on X-ray, may walk with a limp but without apparent pain. Equally, in the same individual, although symptoms may suddenly deteriorate and be associated with a clear cause (such as the development of an effusion, further significant loss of cartilage thickness or collapse of a bony cyst) this is not always the case. Symptomatic or functional deterioration without obvious radiological or clinical changes may occur. Pain and functional impairment remain the best clinical measures of the disease rather than cartilage thickness measurements or chemical tests of cartilage damage (**Table 9.2**).

Table 9.1 Medical approaches to OA.

1 Psychological and social factors

2 Modification of activities of daily living

3 Specific and general exercise programmes

4 Appropriate rest

5 Splints – resting and active

6 Analgesia and NSAIDs

7 Intra-articular corticosteroids

8 Diet and weight loss

9 Complementary approaches

Table 9.2 Differential diagnosis of pain around a joint with mild to moderate radiological OA.

Symptomatic osteoarthritis – local soft tissue problems:

Bursitis
Enthesitis (tender ligament insertions)
Tendonitis
Muscular pain

Pain referred from a proximal site:

Hip pain referred to the knee
Back pain referred to the hip

Pain caused by nerve or nerve root irritation

Coincidental inflammatory arthritis

Generalised pain syndromes:

Fibromyalgia
Polymyalgia rheumatica

Psychological and social factors

Chronic pain and disability have significant psychological and social implications which should not be ignored. Time must be spent listening, assessing the patient's general approach to their pain and relating the presentation to recent major life events. If the pain is long-standing it is reasonable to ask why the patient is presenting now, rather than at some other time. This approach gives the patient permission to open up and speak more generally about themselves. Psychological factors such as depression or anxiety, and social pressures at work or at home naturally affect the patient's ability to cope with his or her problem. Few patients have insight into this. Indeed, the accusatory sentence "Oh, so you just think it is all in my mind" is often a warning sign that there may be more deep-seated problems which need to be addressed. These are sensitive topics and need approaching with sympathy and tact, but the attempt is worthwhile and often leads to better understanding with consequent improvement in quality of life, even if the underlying physical problem remains.

The sense of hopelessness about OA which many patients still describe after seeing a doctor is a sad reflection on the profession's failure to take a more positive approach. One of the aims of this book is to explore just such an approach.

Periarticular soft tissue lesions and joint hyperlaxity

Symptomatic OA should be diagnosed only rarely in patients under 50 years of age. The younger patient is more likely to be suffering pain caused by trauma. Occasionally this will be intra-articular – a haemarthrosis or meniscal tear – but in most it will be a peri-articular lesion of tendon, ligament or bursa. Such lesions may also occur in older patients with mild to moderate radiological OA. They should be specifically sought because they frequently respond to a local steroid injection or physiotherapy and do not necessarily carry the same long-term implications as OA. Direct trauma and 'over-use' injuries are increasing in frequency. If recurrent, they may have serious long-term implications and require expert advice. Their management has been greatly improved by developments in sports medicine which have also encouraged the adoption of more sensible training programmes. Athletes can be difficult to deal with, often expecting unreasonable performance from their bodies and resenting advice about rest or a change of training regime.

It is not clear whether certain sports actually increase the frequency of later OA or simply increase its severity or advance its appearance in susceptible individuals. An additional aspect of later joint OA may be the presence of joint hyperlaxity (*see* **Table 9.3**). Gymnasts and dancers can develop this by training, but during their active period it is often balanced by strong muscles. Later in life, as the muscles become flabby their protective strength is lost, leaving the joint exposed to the risk of abnormal ranges of movement and subsequent articular and peri-articular damage. A small number of individuals show hyperlaxity as part of rare diseases of the connective tissues such as Ehlers–Danlos syndrome or Marfan's syndrome. In the general population there is a spectrum of joint mobility as well as some variation between different racial groups. Such individuals, if recognised early when they present with minor musculoskeletal pains, should be advised by a physiotherapist on how best to protect their joints and spines and be given specific muscle strengthening exercises as a preventative measure.

Primary or secondary OA?

In the younger patient localised or multi-joint OA may be a secondary phenomenon. A consideration of the possible causes of OA occasionally reveals a remediable cause or a problem requiring specialist attention (**Table 9.3**).

Table 9.3 Commoner causes of secondary OA.

Mechanical

Trauma
Previous inflammatory arthritis
Long-leg arthropathy
Hyperlaxity

Congenital

Hip dysplasia
Slipped epiphysis
Legg–Perthe's disease

Systemic Diseases

Acromegaly
Hypothyroidism
Haemochromatosis
Haemophilia
Haemoglobinopathies
Neuropathies

Practical advice for day-to-day life with OA

A balanced attitude to symptomatic OA is important. This depends on the individual and on the specific problem and its severity. The message should never be that nothing can be done, more that nothing need be done in some cases and, in others, that much can be done to make life more tolerable even if some symptoms and disability remain.

Patients should be persuaded to remain as normally active as possible. Undue stressing of the joints will usually be prevented by pain, but tolerable pain can be safely ignored or managed with drugs and does not signify harm. There is little evidence that significant reduction of day-to-day activity will greatly affect the prognosis. When discussing other activities, such as sports or hobbies, their importance to the patient should be balanced against consequent pain and stress on the joints. Sudden-impact stressing and trauma are best avoided and this may mean that some activities such as jogging or heavy manual work should be stopped. The financial implications and retraining difficulties of changing job late in life may make such a suggestion unrealistic, however.

If weight-bearing joints are affected, the patient should walk as desired and necessary, although frequent short walks are preferable to infrequent long hikes. The correct use of a walking stick or sticks of the correct length reduces the weight borne through an affected hip or knee and acts as a useful warning to others of the individual's walking difficulties. Changing to shoes which have a cushioned or shock-absorbent sole and heel may help, as may walking on grass rather than on pavements, although uneven surfaces are a problem, especially for unstable knees. Modifications of the shoe for painful hallux valgus or the trial of a metatarsal bar on the sole for hallux rigidus may also be appropriate.

Rest is helpful during flares of pain and as an adjunct to keeping otherwise normally active. It is probably of more value in inflammatory arthritis, for example, if a joint effusion or acute pseudogout (see below) develops. Individual joints can be rested by the use of a splint.

The value of locally applied heat from a heating pad or hot water bottle is universally recognised and often strikingly demonstrated by the presence of *erythema ab igne*. Similarly, a good soak in a hot bath is soothing. The main effect of heat is to relax painful muscle spasm. Local ice packs help some patients and can be either purchased or adapted from a bag of frozen peas wrapped in a thin towel and moulded to the joint. Ice should not be applied for more than 10 minutes.

Exercises for muscle strength and joint stability

In mild disease, a daily exercise programme should be encouraged. Swimming is an excellent means of maintaining general fitness without stressing weight-bearing joints.

Specific exercises can be isometric or isotonic. During isometric exercise, muscle is strengthened against gravity or resistance with the joint immobile and in its anatomical position. This helps to maintain muscle power and function and is less likely to be inhibited by pain than exercises involving movement. If it is painful the movement should not be against resistance. Specific programmes can be arranged for any affected joint.

How can a physiotherapist help?

Perhaps the most importance role of a physiotherapist in OA is to teach and encourage the patient to exercise, to advise on how best to protect the affected joints by simple modifications of day-to-day activities and, with an occupational therapist, to provide suitable aids and adaptations.

Warm hydrotherapy or spa pools are increasingly available. In weight-bearing joints exercise in warm water relieves pain by a combination of bouyancy and relaxation of painful muscle spasm. A hydrotherapy programme is beneficial just before major joint surgery and during the recovery phase, once the scar has healed. Hydrotherapy can be exhausting for the elderly and is contraindicated in patients with some cardiac problems.

The use of techniques such as ultrasound, diathermy and laser, together with the more traditional treatments with heat and massage are largely empirical and have not been subjected to careful outcome audit. Nonetheless, many patients benefit especially during acute flares of pain. Associated soft-tissue problems may require specific physiotherapeutic treatment. A physiotherapist may help prevent the development of flexion deformities at the hip and knee or correct minor deformities caused by muscle spasm. This preventive role is particularly important after surgery. The objectives of the treatment should be decided by the doctor and therapist jointly and explained to patients so that they have realistic expectations.

Prolonged courses of physiotherapy are unlikely to be cost-effective. The powerful placebo effect of a caring physiotherapist helps the lonely and anxious and may account for requests for prolonged or repeated treatment and lead to inappropriate use of resources.

Drugs in the control of symptomatic OA – a question of risk versus benefit

It is reasonable to tell the patient that the evidence to date suggests that using analgesic and/or anti-inflammatory drugs when necessary does not produce any significant deterioration in OA and may help to retain independence. There is no convincing evidence in clinical trials that non-steroidal anti-inflammatory drugs (NSAIDs) or analgesics themselves either cause OA to deteriorate more rapidly or protect against cartilage damage. Animal models of OA do demonstrate interesting effects with certain drugs but their relevance to human disease remains unclear and claims of 'chondroprotective' actions should be viewed sceptically. The risk of drug side-effects is slight but real and needs to be taken into account, particularly in the elderly. These risks make it necessary to encourage the patient to take drugs only when needed for pain relief and at the lowest effective dose, and to stop taking them from time to time to see whether they are still necessary and beneficial. The use of regular analgesia or NSAIDs over many years without review must be discouraged, although some patients will require regular medication. Drugs are best used in combination with the other therapeutic measures discussed in this chapter.

Analgesics

Patients have often found benefit from simple analgesics such as paracetamol, aspirin or low-dose ibuprofen before they see their doctor. Stronger analgesics containing combinations of paracetamol and codeine or dextropropoxyphene are helpful and may improve sleep if it is disturbed by pain. Side-effects with moderate doses are infrequent, although drowsiness and constipation may be troublesome. Weight-bearing pain is always more difficult to control than resting or night pain.

Non-steroidal anti-inflammatory drugs (NSAIDs)

The value of NSAIDs in the management of painful OA has been clearly established, although their mode of action is uncertain. Their incautious use in the elderly with consequent publicity and the significant risk of gastrointestinal ulceration and consequent bleeding have led to a more circumspect approach to their use. Drug trials have produced a plethora of conflicting results about relative efficacy and safety. The best advice is that the clinician should gain experience with a small selection, which combine low cost with lower than average side-effect profiles as assessed by some of the larger population-based studies. Such a selection might include naproxen, indomethacin, which is cheap but can produce disturbing central side-effects of confusion, unsteadiness or nausea in the elderly, and diclofenac. It is not known why, but different patients benefit differently and it is worth trying several in rotation to find the most suitable. Similarly, if initial benefit is lost, a change may be helpful, assuming that medication is still indicated. Once-daily doses of NSAIDs with a long half-life are convenient, but should be used with great care in the elderly and those with renal or hepatic impairment.

Patients should be forewarned of the commoner side-effects and told what to do should they occur.

Gastrointestinal side-effects

It seems that any of the commonly available NSAIDs can induce gastric erosions and peptic ulceration in susceptible individuals, largely through their suppression of local prostaglandin E_2 synthesis in the gastric mucosa. Prostaglandin E_2 promotes production of bicarbonate and of the protective gastric mucus layer. Soluble or dispersible preparations are less likely to deliver high local concentrations of the drug to the gastric mucosa and rectal administration also reduces the risk. The pro-drugs sulindac and fenbufen are converted to active agents only on the first pass through the liver and so are theoretically less likely to produce direct gastric damage. Nonetheless, blood levels of the active agents, however administered, are still potentially toxic to the mucosa.

Mild and occasional indigestion or heartburn can be treated symptomatically with antacids, but more persistent symptoms should be managed either by changing to a simple analgesic or adding a 4- to 6-week course of an H_2 blocker or synthetic prostaglandin E_2 if the patient is unable to cope without an NSAID. Recurrent symptoms in a patient who needs an NSAID should be investigated by endoscopy rather than barium meal. The relationship between gastric erosions seen on endoscopy, but not visible on barium studies, and the subsequent development of a peptic ulcer is not clear: their presence requires caution. The greatest worry remains the development of acute gastrointestinal bleeding without previous dyspeptic symptoms – a problem with a significant morbidity and mortality in the elderly.

Renal side-effects

Renal blood perfusion is in part dependent on locally produced prostaglandins. This production is impaired by NSAIDs which may therefore adversely affect renal function. Again, the risk is greater in the elderly in whom a pre-treatment and occasional subsequent serum creatinine measurements are warranted. The risk of significant renal problems is increased if NSAIDs are taken in combination with diuretics. Occasionally they can induce an interstitial nephritis. Extreme care should be taken in patients with established renal impairment.

Other side-effects

Asthma may be exacerbated in some patients by the use of NSAIDs, apparently by the induction of an imbalance between the products of the cyclo-oxygenase and the lipoxygenase pathways of arachidonic acid metabolism.

NSAIDs may produce a variety of cutaneous side-effects and patients should be forewarned to stop treatment and seek advice if any develop.

Combinations of analgesics and NSAIDs

The use of combinations of NSAIDs and simple analgesics in more severe pain and whilst a patient is awaiting surgery is acceptable. Other helpful therapy in severe pain may include a sedative or the use of amitriptyline at night which helps some patients by a combination of effects – sedative, antidepressant and analgesic.

Control of synovitis in OA

There is no role for oral or systemic corticosteroids in the management of OA. Despite some reports that intra-articular corticosteroid injections cause deterioration of articular cartilage, especially in weight-bearing joints, the general view is that their occasional use in symptomatic OA is acceptable where an effusion or inflammatory signs indicate that there is synovitis.

Intra-articular corticosteroid injections

When using intra-articular injections it is essential to use a sterile 'no touch' technique, but most clinicians agree that, once learnt under expert supervision, the procedure can be carried out safely in the consulting room and as an outpatient. The most commonly used preparations are microcrystalline hydrocortisone acetate or triamcinolone hexacetonide which remain largely localised to the joint or site of injection. They occasionally cause a 24–48 hour flare of pain which may be severe and about which the patient should be warned. This apart, complications are rare. Superficial injections may lead to marked subcutaneous fat loss and depigmentation of the overlying skin. The dose used for each injection should be varied according to the size of the joint. Any fluid in the joint should be aspirated and it is a wise precaution to send it for bacterial culture. Advise the patient to rest the joint as much as possible for 2 days after the injection, especially if it is a weight-bearing joint, for which a period of bed rest immediately after the injection may improve the response.

CAUTION

Extreme caution should be taken if the joint fluid is cloudy. This may simply reflect an inflammatory component to the disease or the presence of acute pseudogout, but if there is any doubt, the fluid should be examined by Gram staining and cultured to rule out infection before any corticosteroid is introduced. In immunosuppressed patients, those on oral corticosteroids for another disease, and in the very elderly, the intense inflammation and pain typical of an infected joint may be muted. Injection of an infected joint with corticosteroids will usually reduce a rapid flare of pain and, if missed, may lead to severe joint destruction. Any suspected infected joint is a medical emergency requiring immediate specialist attention. Cloudy joint fluid should also be examined under polarised light for crystals implying superimposed gout or pseudogout.

Soft-tissue and peri-articular injections produce symptomatic relief for peri-articular problems such as **de Quervain's tenosynovitis, trochanteric bursitis** or a **tender medial ligament of the knee.**

Diet and OA

There is an association between OA of the knees and obesity in women but it is probable that the obesity is primary rather than secondary to reduced activity. There is little evidence that weight loss has any major effect on OA of weight-bearing joints, but advice to lose weight seems logical and it may delay deterioration and make surgery easier. Weight reduction should be encouraged but not unrealistic expectations of benefit from so doing or the patient will become discouraged and doubtful about further advice.

There is widespread public interest in specific dietary manipulation as a means of controlling disease but only limited scientific evidence of beneficial effects in some cases of arthritis. A multiplicity of different, more or less restrictive dietary regimes is recommended and a variety of dietary supplements is now available, each with its advocates. It cannot be denied that some individuals show apparently dramatic responses, although coincidence and placebo effect may play important roles. Many others try but fail to benefit.

It is best to discuss the approach the patient is interested in to check that the diet is balanced and unlikely to lead to nutritional problems. If necessary a dietician's help should be sought. The use of polyunsaturated oil supplements such as fish oils or evening primrose oil in inflammatory arthritis may have some scientific rationale by changing the nature of some of the pro-inflammatory fatty acid derivatives present in the inflamed synovium and joint effusion. To achieve this effect they need to be taken in high doses, which are expensive, and in combination with a dietary reduction of dairy and meat products in favour of fish and polyunsaturated fats. There is evidence that such an approach may lead to a reduced intake of NSAIDs in some patients with arthritis. Many patients lose weight on such a diet.

Complementary approaches

An increasing public awareness of the potential risks of drug therapy, of its lack of curative actions in arthritis and recent adverse publicity about NSAIDs specifically has led to much greater interest in alternative approaches, both traditional and modern. The medical profession must recognise the limitations of its own therapies and encourage some of this diversity of approach in the interest of its patients and of scientific inquiry. The difficulty in advocating one particular approach over another is that there have been few controlled studies of such alternative approaches and, indeed, it is difficult to see how some could be so studied. A pragmatic view is that, as long as the cost is not prohibitive and there is no apparent risk, patients can be encouraged to try what attracts them. Whatever the method, the power of the placebo in pain management is undeniable and clearly demonstrated in most placebo-controlled drug trials. A highly motivated patient, perhaps encouraged by positive reports from friends, may benefit for a while from homoeopathy, faith healing, acupuncture, reflexology and a vast panoply of more or less exotic methods.

Intractable pain

The important role of surgery in the management of severe pain and disability in OA is discussed in Chapter 11. Osteotomy and excision, interposition or replacement arthroplasty are of increasing importance as materials and techniques improve and complications decrease. Nonetheless, there will always remain a group of patients in whom surgery is not possible for local or general reasons and for whom the level of pain is intolerable. If this is largely pain on movement or weight bearing, the expert advice of an orthotist to provide splints or calipers may be appropriate. In other situations it is better to seek the advice of an occupational therapist on wheelchairs and adaptations to the house to make it more suitable for a chair-bound individuals, or of a social worker on the provision of support services where they are available.

A specialist pain clinic should be considered only when all other approaches have been tried. These clinics use a combination of approaches including regional nerve blocks, transcutaneous nerve stimulation, acupuncture and psychological techniques to help patients to cope better with their pain. A behavioural approach to intractable pain, using psychological and other techniques to improve well-being and promote more normal activity despite the pain will often produce gratifying results. Above all the doctor must try to maintain a positive and practical approach to intractable pain, not promising what it is not possible to deliver but trying to avoid his or her own exasperation in the face of a patient whose whole personality and demeanour have been altered by having to live with pain (**Table 9.4**).

Table 9.4 Approaches to intractable pain caused by OA.

• Surgery

• Regional nerve blocks

• Transcutaneous nerve stimulation

• Acupuncture

• Behavioural means of coping with pain

The management of OA in specific joints

The hand

The hand is the commonest site of radiological OA, affecting more than 50% of the population over the age of 55 years, although only 10% are symptomatic. The combination of Heberden's nodes at the DIP joints and painful, stiff first carpometacarpal joints typical of nodal OA causes inconvenience and considerable anxiety that it may indicate more generalised arthritis. In all patients with nodal OA the risk of more generalised OA is increased but still relatively slight, and need not be mentioned unless the patient specifically asks if it will spread. The knees are the most common additional affected joints in such individuals. Truly generalised OA affecting shoulder, elbow and wrists is rare, although more common if there is coexistent generalised chondrocalcinosis (see below).

Symptomatic OA of the hand

The Heberden' node (**9.1**) is the most typical feature of nodal OA and the commonest marker of the slightly increased risk of OA of the knees or of generalised OA. In the early phase of their development, Heberden's nodes may be painful, with joint redness and swelling suggesting that, at least in some, the onset of this so-called 'degenerative' arthritis is inflammatory in nature. Similar acutely painful episodes may occur during the development of early OA of the PIP joints and at the first CMC joint. The best management is to reassure the patient that these episodes are short-lived (a matter of weeks or a few months in most) and will resolve with reduction of pain, although bony swelling and some deformity may develop and remain.

9.1

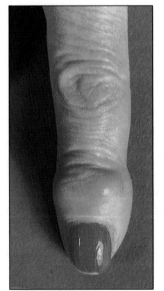

9.1 Nodal OA of the hand – a Heberden's node.

Involvement of the proximal interphalangeal joints (**9.2**) in nodal OA, particularly during the inflammatory stage and/or when the DIP joints are not affected, is occasionally misinterpreted as rheumatoid arthritis. A weakly positive rheumatoid factor is commonly found in the older patient and this merely compounds the problem. If the hand alone is involved the differential diagnosis does not affect the treatment, which is with simple analgesics or with NSAIDs, depending on the severity of any pain or stiffness. The prognosis is, however, significantly different and an incorrect diagnosis of rheumatoid arthritis will cause unnecessary anxiety. Severe morning stiffness, swelling of other joints and a raised ESR may be indicators that it is indeed rheumatoid arthritis.

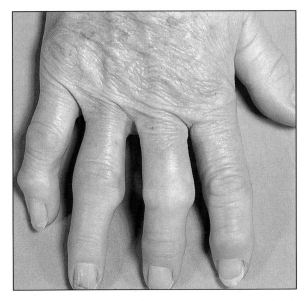

9.2 Nodal OA – Bouchard's nodes.

Persistent pain from chronic first CMC joint OA is not uncommon and may be the most troublesome aspect of the disease in the hand. It makes gripping and squeezing difficult. There is associated localised first CMC joint tenderness and pain and crepitus on manipulation. In most patients the pain settles and the joint stiffens as time passes, leaving the typical squared hand of OA caused by adduction of the first metacarpal (**9.3**). This is not disabling, except that it reduces the span.

Some patients with persistent pain are helped by a splint which encircles the base of the thumb and the wrist, effectively immobilising the first CMC joint alone. Some patients will not tolerate the inconvenience of such a splint.

Not all patients experience acute painful episodes. If the fingers are painless nothing need be done except to encourage using the hand as normally as possible. It is sensible to use aids to open tight jars and bottles and avoid undue stress to the base of the thumb from carrying heavy trays or pans.

Hot wax baths are a traditional and comforting method of treating painful and stiff hands, but afford little long-term benefit. The use of hot wax at home should be discouraged because of the risks of accidental burning. Exercising the hands every morning by squeezing a sponge rhythmically in hot water is comforting and safer and will help to maintain mobility.

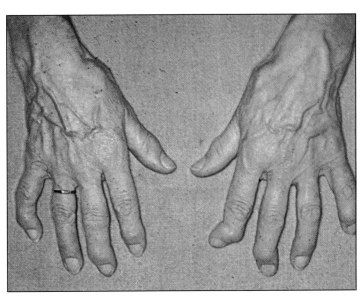

9.3 First carpometacarpal OA – the 'square' hand.

Oral analgesics or NSAIDs are rarely indicated for symptomatic OA limited to the hands. Gels which contain NSAIDs for local application are of limited benefit for large joints and deep structures, but their use in these superficially sited joints helps some patients during the acute phase. If the pain is intolerable some advocate the use of small doses of intra-articular steroids. The procedure has a greater place in the management of painful first CMC joints than in the DIP or PIP joints; a fine needle should be used. Patients should be warned that it is not always helpful and may increase the pain for a few days.

In a few patients the pain persists and surgery is indicated. A painful and unstable thumb IP joint can be simply fused with great functional benefit. In a few individuals persistent first CMC joint pain can be helped by replacement arthroplasty.

Peri-articular problems in the hand

First CMC joint OA must be distinguished from **de Quervain's tenosynovitis**; forced flexion of the thumb into the palm (Finkelstein's test) causes pain in both conditions, but in de Quervain's the pain is mainly felt over the radial styloid where there is localised swelling and tenderness, rather than over the first CMC joint itself as in OA. **Nodular flexor tenosynovitis** may produce painful stiffening of the finger and occasionally a trigger finger. The nodules are usually palpable over the palmar aspect of the metacarpal bone or the proximal phalanx and will usually respond to a local corticosteroid injection.

The knee

Unilateral and unicompartmental OA of the knee are common sequelae to earlier injury, particularly meniscal tears. It seems likely that it is trauma in combination with a hereditary tendency which determines whether an individual will develop this complication in later life; not all do. Early surgical management of the tear does not seem to affect the eventual development of OA although partial meniscectomy is preferable when feasible.

Symptomatic OA of the knee

Mild pain associated with mild or moderate radiological OA and minimal or absent deformity is often helped by non-weight-bearing quadriceps-strengthening exercises. Exercises should be continued, even if the pain worsens, as a preventive measure. The quadriceps mechanism is essential to the stability and function of the knee through its action on the patella. Simple quadriceps exercises for osteoarthritic knees can be taught without referral to a physiotherapist if the patient is well motivated.

QUADRICEPS EXERCISES

Instruct the patient to lie with a small rolled towel behind the knees. The exercise consists of first straightening one knee and then dorsiflexing and internally rotating the foot before finally lifting the straight leg slightly and holding it for a while, gradually increasing the period as stamina improves.

Repeat with alternate knees several times.

For isotonic exercises for the quadriceps, the patient sits slightly reclining, with the back supported and the leg hanging free at the knee. The knee is straightened, initially against gravity alone and then, if possible, with a 1/2–2 kg weight added at the ankle. There is evidence that an effusion in the knee produces reflex inhibition of maximum voluntary quadriceps contraction when compared with that elicited by external stimulation. In such circumstances draining the effusion and the injection of a small dose of corticosteroid should be considered.

Although analgesics and/or NSAIDs may be of value the effect is often limited to reducing rest and night pain. Weight-bearing pain and especially the pain of the first few steps after sitting or in the morning are more difficult to control and the patient may have to be encouraged to understand this and learn to cope with it. Avoiding sitting immobile for long periods is helpful but makes such activities as visiting the theatre a problem.

During acute exacerbations, especially when there is an effusion, aspiration and injection of steroids can be considered but should not be performed too often; preferably not more than twice a year. In the presence of tibial plateau collapse intra-articular steroids are best avoided as they may cause further rapid bone loss. The knee is the second commonest site, after the wrist, for developing **acute pseudogout** (see below).

Once it is clear that the problem is progressive and disabling, that deformity is developing (typically a varus deformity as shown in **9.4**, caused by medial compartment OA), and that pain is poorly controlled and sleep disturbed, the advice of an orthopaedic surgeon with an interest in surgery of the knee should be sought. The choice will lie between osteotomy in unicompartment disease, or surface or total joint replacement arthroplasty. The outcome of knee replacement surgery is improving all the time but still remains less predictable than that of the total hip replacement, largely because of the slightly increased risks of peri-operative infection and of later loosening. As with all surgery, the patient must be made aware of what can be expected from the operation and what the risks and limitations of the procedure are likely to be.

9.4

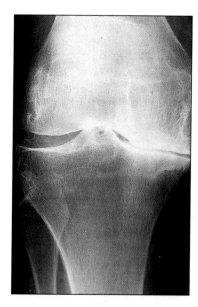

9.4 Radiograph of severe deforming OA of the knee.

In the patient who is inoperable for reasons of general health the use of a hinged collateral knee support splint may be helpful to improve mobility, especially if the knee joint shows collateral instability. Such splints are, however, cumbersome and unsightly. Sticks or crutches may help mobility to a limited extent. If a wheelchair is resorted to it is essential to avoid the development of fixed flexion deformities of both hip and knee by active and passive exercises and brief periods of lying prone.

Peri-articular knee problems

Minor radiological OA of the knees in the middle-aged and elderly is common. Small marginal osteophytes and minimal joint space narrowing are of no significance and other causes of knee pain should be sought. **Medial or lateral collateral ligament strains** cause local tenderness at their points of insertion into the tibia. **Anserine bursitis** causes tenderness over the anteromedial border of the upper tibia at the site of insertion of the tendon of sartorius. It particularly affects obese women. Peripatellar pain may be caused by **pre-** or **infrapatellar bursitis** or arises at the insertion of the quadriceps or the patellar tendon into the patella. These are all best treated with a local corticosteroid injection or with physiotherapy, depending on their severity. Once the pain has settled, graded quadriceps exercises should be encouraged.

The hip

Hip OA typically produces weight-bearing pain in the groin and buttock radiating down the front of the thigh to the knee, although it may be localised to the thigh and/or knee. There is usually associated stiffness which makes it difficult to reach the foot to cut toe nails or put on shoes on the affected side.

Symptomatic hip OA

Although analgesics and/or NSAIDs may be of value, the effect is often limited to reducing rest and night pain. Weight-bearing pain and especially the pain of the first few steps after sitting are more difficult to help and the patient may have to be encouraged to cope with this. Patients should avoid sitting immobile for long periods, and should be encouraged to remain as mobile as possible, using a stick if necessary. They should also lose weight, especially if surgery is contemplated (**9.5**).

9.5

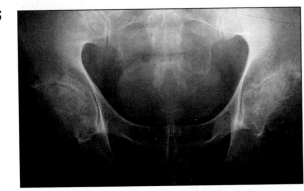

9.5 Radiograph of severe OA of the hips.

Although not inevitably, most patients will eventually need referral for a total hip replacement. The operation is now generally highly successful although it is essential that the patient is counselled about what to expect in the immediate and longer term. In the younger patient surgery should be avoided for as long as reasonably possible because of the likely need for re-replacement after between 5 and 15 years. In a few patient osteotomy helps for a while. Nonetheless, it is now clear that, despite the possible need for reoperation after a number of years because of loosening, replacement surgery should be undertaken even in the younger patient once it is clear that the pain is intolerable and disabling.

Aspiration and intra-articular injection of the hip is technically difficult and should be performed by an expert. It has some value in acute exacerbations. Whether it significantly increases the risk of aseptic necrosis is not clear.

Peri-articular hip problems

As with the knee, the hip X-ray may show minor peri-articular osteophytes and minor joint space narrowing without producing symptoms. Associated 'hip' pain should be more carefully defined, as the word hip is relatively nonspecific and used by the public to describe a wide area from the iliac crest to the greater trochanter. Tender **fibrositic nodules** lying over the upper buttocks may produce pain radiating into the buttock and down the posterolateral thigh and will often respond to a local injection of corticosteroid. **Trochanteric bursitis** produces pain over the trochanter and outer thigh which is worse on walking, on climbing stairs and when lying on the affected side, and is associated with localised tenderness overlying or just proximal to the greater trochanter. It may coexist with symptomatic OA and will often respond to local corticosteroid. The burning dysaesthesiae and pain over the anterolateral thigh caused by **meralgia paraesthetica** is occasionally mistaken for symptomatic OA of the hip. Pain in the upper leg or buttock may be referred from the back.

First MTP/bunion

The commonest cause of pain in the great toe is pressure from ill-fitting shoes. With time, the development of a valgus deformity at the MTP joint (**9.6**) leads to increased pressure over the medial aspect of the joint and in turn to development of an adventitious bursa or bunion. Chronic inflammation and occasional ulceration can generally be reduced by padding and careful attention to shoe wear, avoiding tight, pointed shoes and seams running over the pressure point.

In some the great toe MTP joint becomes stiff and painful due to loss of joint space and periarticular osteophytes; true OA leading to hallux rigidus (**9.7**). If the condition is mild, cushion-soled shoes may be sufficient. A few patients learn to wear a metatarsal rocker bar on the sole of the shoe which permits the foot to rock during walking without requiring the toe to flex. If pain is intolerable, excision arthroplasty is probably the most helpful procedure, combined with a realignment procedure if there is significant hallux valgus.

9.6

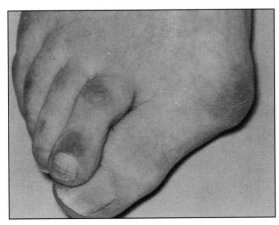

9.6 Hallux valgus .

9.7

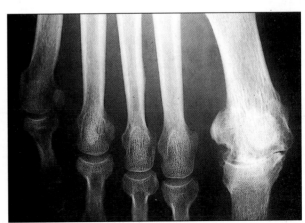

9.7 Radiograph showing hallux rigidus

Chondrocalcinosis and acute pseudogout

Radiological evidence of chondrocalcinosis increases in frequency with increasing age, reaching an incidence of more than 5% in those aged over 70 years. In most it is an asymptomatic finding. It may be associated with **pseudo-osteoarthritis** which affects a different pattern of joints – knees, wrists, MCPs, hips and shoulders, and about 5% of patients with widespread chondrocalcinosis have an inflammatory arthritis which mimics rheumatoid arthritis.

One in four patients with chondrocalcinosis develops episodic acute inflammatory arthritis which mimics acute urate gout except that it more commonly affects the wrists and knees and may be polyarticular. In the wrist chondrocalcinosis is most easily seen in the triangular ligament (**9.8**). In the knee it may be seen in the fibrocartilages or menisci. This is best seen on the anteroposterior X-ray (**9.9**) as an irregular triangular shape between the femoral condyles and the tibial plateaux, while that of the hyaline cartilage is best seen in lateral view as a line of calcification parallel to the surface of the femur (**9.10**). In this advanced case hyaline chondrocalcinosis is also clearly seen in the anteroposterior view in the lateral compartment. This patient, as well as experiencing attacks of acute pseudogout, shows secondary OA of the knee on X-ray and had the typical symptoms of weight-bearing pain and gelling after immobility between the acute attacks.

9.8

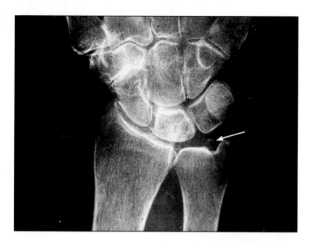

9.8–9.10 Radiograph showing chondrocalcinosis of wrist and knee.

9.9

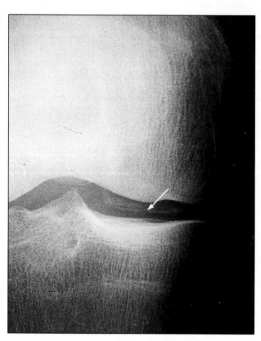

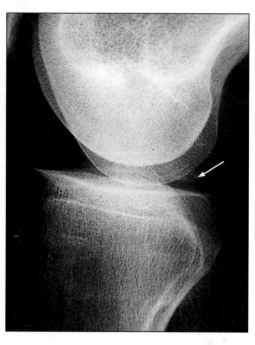

9.10

Examination of the joint fluid reveals rhomboidal, weakly positively birefringent intracellular and extracellular crystals of calcium pyrophosphate (**9.11**). The cause of shedding of the crystals of calcium pyrophosphate into the joint is not known, nor do they always cause acute inflammation. The attacks may be precipitated by surgery or an acute illness. The acute inflammatory arthritis lasts about two weeks if untreated and may be associated with fever and a leucocytosis; infective arthritis is an important differential diagnosis. Occasionally gout occurs coincidentally and can be recognised by the presence of needle-shaped, strongly negatively birefringent crystals of sodium urate.

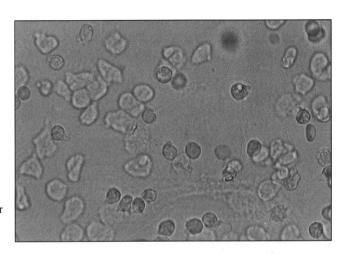

9.11

9.11 Calcium pyrophosphate crystals seen under polarised light.

Acute pseudogout responds well to therapeutic aspiration of the joint combined with the use of NSAIDs in initially high doses. Colchicine is also effective and safer in patients with a history of peptic ulceration. In a very painful joint a local or intramuscular corticosteroid injection can be used if infection can be safely discounted. In recurrent attacks repeated aspiration is not necessary unless drug therapy is unsuccessful. Occasionally prophylactic doses of an NSAID or of colchine may be needed. Allopurinol is ineffective.

Chondrocalcinosis appearing in a patient under 50 years of age may indicate a variety of predisposing metabolic diseases, including hyperparathyroidism, haemochromatosis, hypomagnesaemia and hypophosphatasia (see Chapter 7).

Fibromyalgia

Patients with fibromyalgia (often, but not exclusively, middle-aged and energetic women) can present with an exasperating battery of complaints. To the rheumatologist they complain of 'pain all over', to the neurologist of typical tension headaches and to the gastroenterologist of the myriad symptoms of irritable bowel syndrome. The patients with predominantly rheumatological symptoms frequently complain bitterly of long-standing and widespread pain not helped by a wide variety of drugs and physical techniques which they have already tried. To this is added the exasperation of finding that doctors can find nothing wrong on numerous tests, while X-rays show minimal OA changes or spondylosis, which are sometimes and erroneously used to dismiss the problem in terms of 'wear and tear'. The patients are often introspective and anxious about a variety of things but with little insight. They are usually unprepared to conceive that anxiety and stress can play a role in their symptoms. Such patients are demanding of a doctor's time and expect consistent explanations which *they* find acceptable to account for their symptoms – the rheumatological 'heart sink' patient. Although it is, of course, necessary to exclude serious pathology, the length of time that the symptoms have been present and the patient's ability to carry on despite them are important clues. Indeed, this very drive to carry on with a busy life despite the pain often brings powerful reinforcement by being thought of as 'brave' or 'remarkable' by doting friends and family. Sleep is usually disturbed and typically unsatisfying with the patient wakening unrefreshed.

Fibromyalgia is an important and useful diagnosis. It recognises that the one typical unifying feature of these patients is the presence of surprisingly tender and well-defined trigger points. A variety of different points has been described. The exact number and location may not be as important as the fact that they all represent areas of the body which are to some extent tender in all but which are markedly so in these patients. Not only is the finding of these trigger points of diagnostic significance but it often comes as a surprise to the patient, who may not have found them herself and who is grateful that, at last, something abnormal has been found.

The management of these patients is complex and tiring. Reassurance that the pain can be explained and is not caused by some fatal or potentially disabling disease is gratefully received, but usually tempered by the fact that the syndrome itself is difficult to relieve. The trigger points are generally over muscular insertions into bone, but only occasionally helped by local injections. There are no clear descriptions of abnormal pathology either at these sites or in the muscles. Reflex muscle spasm, increased awareness of normal or slightly increased sensory activity and a pattern of pain, itself inducing painful muscle spasm to create a vicious circle are concepts which can be used to explain the syndrome.

Graded exercise programmes and hydrotherapy may be helpful particularly if the patient is generally unfit. Relaxation, yoga and massage help some. Although analgesics and anti-inflammatory drugs are rarely helpful, they might be tried for brief periods in an attempt to break the pain circle. Amitriptyline used at night also helps some individuals, probably by restoring a more normal sleep pattern. Although this drug may also help if the patient is depressed, it is wise to stress that it is not being used primarily as an antidepressant or there is a risk of alienating the patient. Although often difficult and demanding, such patients are genuinely in trouble and deserve reassurance and help despite the limitations of present understanding both about the pathological problem and its control.

Conclusion

Radiological OA is too often used to explain articular or peri-articular pain without proper examination or thought and with the implication that, being caused by wear and tear, nothing can be done. This approach reinforces the popular view that any form of arthritis has an inevitably bad prognosis. Local peri-articular problems should be treated. If symptoms remain and are clearly caused by symptomatic OA, although it is technically 'incurable', it should be discussed with the patient positively in terms of what can be done to help and of the likely prognosis, which is often not as bad as the individual may fear. Explanation and reassurance will help patients to cope better with episodic flares and a sympathetic discussion of the availability of surgery if the situation becomes intolerable should also give reassurance. Many patients will admit that they can cope with their present pain and disability but are scared about the likely outcome, a fear often engendered by a relative or acquaintance who has been badly disabled in the past.

10. Chondroprotection and Models of Osteoarthritis

Adrian Jones; Joanna Ledingham; Michael Doherty

Osteoarthritis as a process that can be manipulated

As discussed in other chapters, osteoarthritis (OA) is not a simple 'wear and tear' phenomenon but an active process (**10.1**) which is part of the reparative response to injury. It is reasonable, therefore, to postulate that such a process might be manipulated to produce beneficial or detrimental effects on joint function and symptoms. This has led to the current interest in 'chondroprotective agents' (CPAs) and 'chondrodestructive' agents whose use may beneficially or adversely affect the OA process. The use of 'chondro' to describe such agents reflects the current emphasis on cartilage. This may not be totally appropriate (Doherty, 1989).

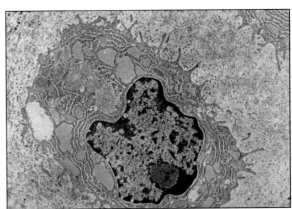

10.1

10.1 Electron micrograph of a chondrocyte from an osteoarthritic joint demonstrating marked biosynthetic activity.

Chondroprotection or arthroprotection?

Joints are complex organs (**10.2**) and their successful function is not simply the result of a single tissue, i.e. articular cartilage. It is possible to have a fully functional joint in the absence of cartilage (**10.3, 10.4**). Other tissues may be equally important and indeed may, in terms of symptoms, be more so (**10.5**). Drugs can also have important effects on these tissues. A well-described example is the effect non-steroidal anti-inflammatory drugs (NSAIDs) can have on bone at standard pharmacological doses; heterotopic ossification following hip replacement surgery (**10.6**) can be prevented by NSAIDs including indomethacin (Ritter and Gioe, 1982). While it is not clear whether such an effect would be adaptive or maladaptive in OA, the danger of extrapolating from effects on single tissues is clear. It would perhaps be better to use the terms 'arthroprotective' and 'arthrodestructive' to emphasise the need to concentrate on the functioning of the total joint rather than a single component.

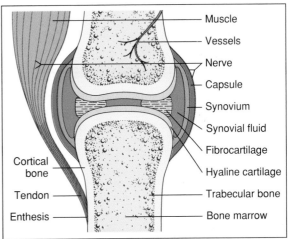

10.2

Muscle
Vessels
Nerve
Capsule
Synovium
Synovial fluid
Fibrocartilage
Hyaline cartilage
Trabecular bone
Bone marrow

Cortical bone
Tendon
Enthesis

10.2 The synovial joint is a complex structure requiring many tissues for successful, normal function.

10.3 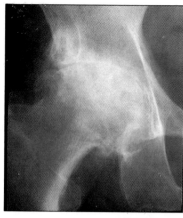 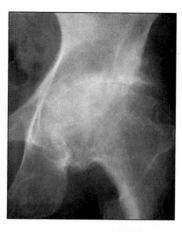 **10.4**

10.3, 10.4 In spite of marked, bilateral joint space loss this 68-year-old man was asymptomatic and though he had limitation of hip movement experienced no handicap.

10.5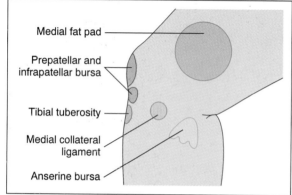

Medial fat pad

Prepatellar and infrapatellar bursa

Tibial tuberosity

Medial collateral ligament

Anserine bursa

10.5 Many structures around a synovial joint may give rise to symptoms as illustrated here in the case of the medial aspect of the knee.

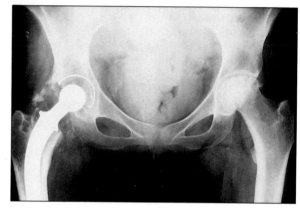 10

10.6 Heterotopic ossification following total hip replacement.

Studying chondroprotection

As will be discussed later, the study of chondroprotection in spontaneous human OA is difficult. Much of the available data are thus derived from laboratory evidence. Several experimental methods for studying OA are available: *in vitro* biochemical assays; *ex vivo* effects in cell and organ culture; and in vivo animal models. Each of these will be discussed in turn, followed by a discussion of the available human data.

Biochemical actions of putative CPAs

Several biochemical and cellular mechanisms are thought to be involved in cartilage degradation in OA (**10.7**; Chapter 3). It might therefore be supposed that pharmacological agents which can interfere with these processes could be beneficial or detrimental in OA. Whilst this approach may identify candidate CPAs for future study, there are many inherent difficulties which largely result from the complex nature of the mechanisms involved. Thus, although this approach has been used for the development of, for example, specific enzyme inhibitors that might delay tissue degradation, it has not been extensively used.

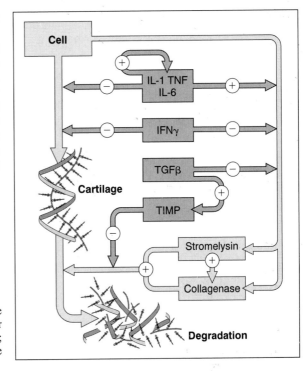

10.7 Biochemical and cellular mechanisms of cartilage synthesis and degradation. (IL-1, interleukin 1; TNF, tumour necrosis factor; IL-6, interleukin 6; IFN, interferon gamma; TGF, transforming growth factor beta; TIMP, tissue inhibitors of metalloproteinases; 1 stimulates; 2 inhibits.)

Ex vivo experiments

Many of the objections relating to isolating and studying individual biochemical mechanisms can be overcome by the use of cell, tissue or organ culture (e.g. see Burkhardt and Ghosh, 1987). There are, however, still many problems inherent in such an approach.

- **The mechanisms involved are not yet well understood.** Thus accurate recreation of *in vivo* conditions *ex vivo* is difficult. Indeed, cellular and tissue behaviour may be affected by experimental conditions.
- **The systems of repair and degradation are inextricably linked.** Conditions *ex vivo* may not preserve this linkage nor may we be able to distinguish which processes are involved in a given outcome. For example, enzyme degradation may be an essential component of remodelling and repair.
- **The source of the experimental tissue may be important,** e.g. differences between species, donor age and site of origin. Chondrocytes appear to demonstrate marked biological variability, even

from different areas within the same cartilage sample.
- **There may be an undue emphasis on a single tissue,** cartilage in particular.
- **CPA concentrations *in vivo* and access to tissues may be very different *ex vivo*.** This may be particularly important if other tissues are important in producing active metabolites of CPAs.
- **The correlations between cellular, tissue and organ process and the clinical syndrome of OA are unknown.** Extrapolation of results is thus difficult.

However, data derived from such experiments do support the notion that drugs could be potentially beneficial or detrimental to the OA process (**Table 10.1**). Such effects can be measured by demonstrating potentially beneficial effects on cartilage biochemistry or chondrocyte cytomorphology (**10.8**). Such experiments might be used as a preliminary method for identifying putative CPAs.

10.8

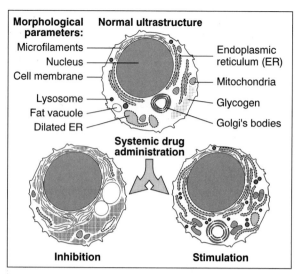

10.8 Annesley chondrocyte morphology assay (Reproduced with kind permission from *Int. J. Tissue Reaction* 1985, **7**, 273–289.)

Table 10.1 Data derived in *in vitro* systems for the action of certain pharmacological agents (Sa, salicylate; In, indomethacin; TA, tiaprofenic acid; Dc, diclofenac; St, corticosteroid; SPP, sodium pentosan polyphosphate; GAG-PS, glycosaminoglycans polysulphate; GP-C, glycosaminoglycans-peptide complex; PG, proteoglycan; HA, hyaluronic acid; HAase, hyaluronidase: −, potentially pro-arthritic; +, anti-arthritic; 0, no effect)

	Sa	In	TA	Dc	St	SPP	GAG-PS	GP-C
PG synthesis	−	0/−	0/+	0	−		+	+
HA synthesis			+/−	+	+		+	
Protein synthesis	−	−					+	+
Chondrocyte morphology	−	+			−			
PG degradation	0/+	0	0/+		0/+	+	+	+
HAase						+	+	+
Elastase				+		+	+	+
Collagenase	+		+	+		+	+	+
'Catabolic' factors	+	+		+	+			
Complement activity						+		
Prostaglandin synthesis	+	+	+	+	+		+	
Oxygen derived free radicals				+				

Chondroprotection in animals

Validity of the models

Some of the objections related to *in vitro* and *ex vivo* models are overcome by the use of whole animal models. In particular, the response of the entire joint to damage can be assessed. There are however a number of remaining, possibly insurmountable problems relating to their relevance to human OA (Troyer, 1982):

- There may be significant interspecies variation in joint response.
- The mechanism of initiation of the 'OA' process may not replicate human disease; many models use different physical and chemical joint insults (**10.9**) and whilst this may produce a joint response, this may not mirror 'spontaneous' human OA.

- The experimental response may involve short-term effects on joints which may not be representative of established human OA. For example, in the Pond-Nuki model of dog OA (the response to section of the anterior cruciate ligament) often only early changes are studied in which marked cartilage hypertrophy is observed rather than cartilage destruction, which is the feature of established human disease.
- There may still be an undue over-emphasis on a single tissue, in particular, cartilage.
- The correlations between structural change and the clinical syndrome of human OA are unknown; therefore although a structural effect is observed it may not be clear whether this is an adaptive or maladaptive response, nor can symptoms be adequately assessed.

Nevertheless, although it is necessary to be wary of extrapolating animal data to humans, these models do provide a means of elucidating some of the mechanisms involved in OA, and evidence for a possible modulating effect of drugs.

10.9

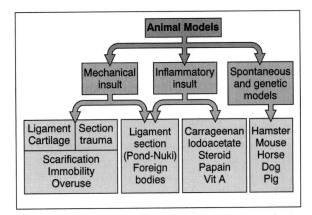

10.9 Animal models of 'osteoarthritis'.

Chondroprotection in animal models

Some purative CPAs, and potentially chondrodestructive drugs, have been assessed in animal test systems. A number of such studies are summarised (**Table 10.2**). As can be seen, although there is broad agreement in the data there are conflicting results. This may arise from inter-species variation as well as methodological differences. Ultimately only human studies can resolve the issue as to whether these drugs will be of benefit in the human situation.

Table 10.2 Actions of pharmacological agents in animal models of OA (Sa, salicylate; In, indomethacin; TA, tiaprofenic acid; Dc, diclofenac; St, corticosteroid; SPP, sodium pentosan polyphosphate; GAG-PS, glycosaminoglycans polysulphate; GP-C, glycosaminoglycans-peptide complex; PG, proteoglycan; Tr, tribenoside; + anti-arthrogenic; − proarthrogenic; 0, no effect).

	Sa	In	Dc	TA	St	SPP	GAG-PS	GP-C	Tr
Chicken	−	−	0	0	−	+	+	+	+
Mouse	−	−	+	0/+	−		+	+	+
Rat	−	−	+/−	+/−	−		+		
Rabbit	0	0/−	+/−	+/−	+/−	+	+	+	+
Dog	−	0/−	0	0/+	+		+	+	

How can we assess chondroprotection in humans?

Although some studies have attempted to determine whether drugs affect human OA, part of the reason the results remain controversial is because of the difficulty in assessing any arthroprotective or arthrodestructive effect. Many methods exist to assess OA, but all are flawed by an inability to define the condition precisely (Dieppe, 1990). As has long been noted, there can be a marked discordance between symptoms and structural change (**10.10**) and thus the condition may be viewed quite differently by the clinician, biochemist, anatomist and, most importantly, the patient.

The chief aspect of OA which confronts the patient is pain. Thus symptomatic response has always been fundamental in assessing therapeutic response. However, symptoms may show short-term fluctuations or even resolve (**10.11**), whereas structural change tends to be slower. It is thus difficult to know whether short-term symptom response and long-term structural and functional outcome are related. It is possible that an initial symptomatic deterioration, e.g. synovitis, may produce the conditions necessary for a long-term beneficial outcome.

Two broad approaches have been used to try to examine the underlying structural and physicochemical aspects of the OA process: radiographic imaging and biochemical markers of joint metabolism.

10.10

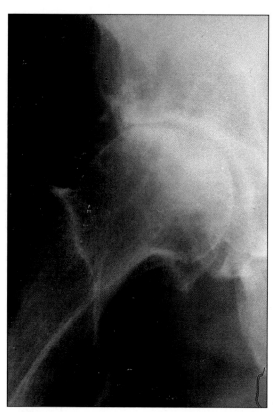

10.10 Despite severe structural damage this patient was entirely asymptomatic apart from a moderate restriction of hip movement.

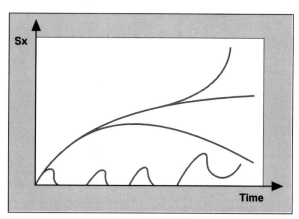

10.11 Symptoms may be episodic, progressive, remit, or plateau with time.

Radiographic assessment

Radiology is used as a substitute for anatomy. In addition, there have also been attempts to use radiographs to quantify structural change. The commonest grading system in use is that of Kellgren and Lawrence (1957) (**10.12**). It has been suggested that it is possible to use such a semi-quantitive system to assess the response of OA joints to CPAs. There are a few problems, however, with such an approach, as can be illustrated by reference to the Kellgren and Lawrence grading system (KLGS).

• Not all features assessed may be relevant. For example, osteophytes are given a prominent place in the KLGS, however their importance in OA is debatable; they may in fact be a beneficial remodelling response to abnormal loading.

• The system may not be hierarchical and different radiographic features may represent different aspects of the OA process. For example, in atrophic OA it may be possible to have severe joint space loss without osteophyte formation.

• The grading may be too crude. The KLGS has only four possible grades and thus subtle changes will be difficult if not impossible to measure. This is particularly important if chondroprotection is to be measured within a reasonable time-scale.

• Parameters may not be reproducibly assessed. Not only may inter-observer and intra-observer variability be important, but also the method of measurement may have an important bearing on the results obtained. For example, in the study by Rashad *et al.* (1989), discussed later in this chapter, because loss of joint space in one part of the hip joint can produce paradoxical widening at other sites (**10.13**), combining measurements from different sites produces a meaningless measure of cartilage loss.

• Radiographic change is a record of past physiological response. Radiology provides a poor indication of when and how structural change occurred. In particular, there is no information as to whether the OA process is still active or likely to progress.

In order to overcome these problems a number of refinements can be made, for example independent scoring of various parameters or automated image analysis. Even then, however, one fundamental problem remains: radiographs reliably detect only bony changes. Cadaveric studies demonstrate that severe OA changes can be present in the absence of radiographic change (Dieppe 1990). The use of other methods of imaging has thus been explored.

Radionuclide imaging is dependent on physiological changes in vasculature and mineralization. At least some of these abnormalities have been shown to be predictive of outcome (Hutton *et al.*, 1986). In future it may be possible to determine if CPAs can affect scintigraphic appearance in a way that might be of benefit for joint outcome (**10.14**).

Magnetic resonance imaging, a newer technique, may also have an important role to play. Not only can cartilage and soft tissues be imaged, but some physiological parameters can also be assessed (**10.15**). There may, however, be problems of spatial resolution.

Regardless of any future role for these techniques, long-term, prospective studies are still required to determine whether the changes that are seen have important practical as opposed to theoretical influences on outcome.

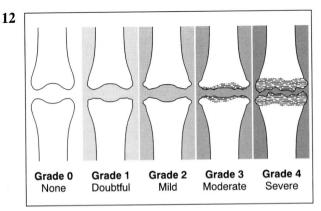

10.12 The basis of the Kellgren and Lawrence grading system of OA, which is based on osteophytosis, joint space loss and subchondral bone changes.

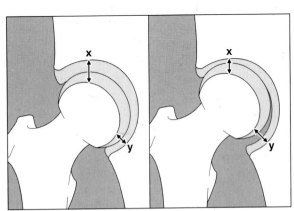

10.13 The problem with the scoring system for joint space loss used by Rashad *et al.*, whereby loss in one portion of the joint may produce apparent widening at another site.

10.14

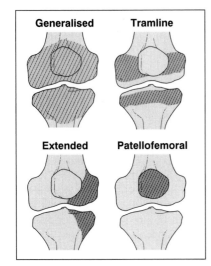

Generalised   Tramline

Extended   Patellofemoral

10.15

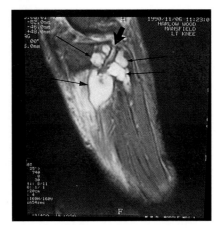

10.14 The four basic scintigraphic appearances that may be observed in osteoarthritis.

10.15 A coronal magnetic resonance image of the superior tibiofibular and lateral tibio-femoral joints demonstrating joint space narrowing and marked cystic change.

Biochemical markers

In the same way that measurement of hydroxyproline excretion and alkaline phosphatase allows assessment of activity of Paget's disease, it has been hoped that similar markers of cartilage and bone turnover might also be of use in OA; many of these have already been discussed (*see* Chapter 3). Although many putative markers have been investigated there are some inherent problems in this approach (Brandt, 1989):

- The normal physiology of many markers is unknown. Short-term fluctuations in marker molecules may not be caused by changes in the OA process. Similarly, drugs might have effects on marker metabolism independent of effects on OA metabolism; for example, by altering synovial permeability, or renal or hepatic clearance.
- Markers arise from more than one joint. This is a particular problem in assessing the response to local therapy. It is also a problem if differing disease processes result in marker release from different sites, for example the patient with post-meniscectomy knee OA who also has cervical spondylosis and gout. Measuring local marker concentrations in synovial fluid only partially overcomes this problem: such fluid may be difficult to obtain; differing intra-articular volumes may make turnover difficult to assess; and normal values are largely unknown.
- Marker turnover is dependent on the amount of active tissue (**10.16**). As OA progresses the amount of metabolically active cartilage and bone able to synthesise marker molecules will probably vary considerably. Differentiating tissue mass from tissue activity may prove extremely difficult.
- No single marker may reflect the OA process. The OA process probably comprises several aspects including: initiating events, adaptive response, and perpetuating processes. There is also a balance of synthesis and degradation. Understanding which markers reflect which aspects of the OA process and indeed which processes are beneficial or detrimental is difficult, but will be crucial if markers are to be of value in assessing OA.

10.16

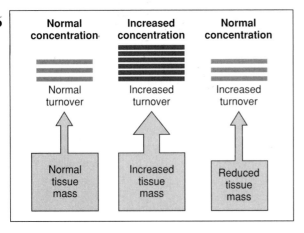

Normal concentration	Increased concentration	Normal concentration
Normal turnover	Increased turnover	Increased turnover
Normal tissue mass	Increased tissue mass	Reduced tissue mass

10.16 Marker concentrations observed in body fluids depend on both the amount of 'source' tissue as well as the rate at which it is being turned over.

Ultimately the value of CPAs will have to be assessed in terms of patient benefit, i.e. in terms of maintenance and restoration of function and relief of symptoms. Whilst other means of assessment may aid the identification of promising CPAs and their mechanisms of action, long-term clinical trials are paramount in establishing their claim to be chondroprotective. In addition to assessment, a number of problems are inherent in such trials which relate primarily to problems of blinding and long-term compliance. They also require substantial investment of time and resources if they are to be conducted efficiently. Currently such studies have looked only at established OA, and it is possible that greater benefit would result if early OA was studied. However, at present there is no way of identifying early OA.

Two methods may allow this. First, patients with OA at one site slowly accrue OA at other sites. This rate of acquisition of new sites might be a parameter that would be affected by CPAs (Dieppe, 1990). These new sites, however, are likely to represent established, but non-detectable OA. Second, OA may develop in predisposed individuals who undergo meniscectomy (Doherty et al, 1983). Although prophylactic intervention at this stage would require longer-term follow-up to establish a chondroprotective effect, this might be a model in which to test CPAs in unestablished OA.

Drugs and adverse effects on the OA process

OA is common and therefore there may already be evidence that currently available drugs can adversely or beneficially affect it. Two major groups of drugs have been examined: non-steroidal anti-inflammatory drugs (NSAIDs) and corticosteroids.

Does 'Indocid hip' exist?

In 1967 Coke presented a series of 24 patients treated with indomethacin. In the ensuing discussion it was pointed out that some patients had developed a rapidly destructive hip arthropathy. Since then a number of cases and series have been reported of a similar destructive arthropathy occurring in patients receiving NSAIDs (**10.17**). However, as Coke was first to point out, such changes may also be seen in patients not receiving NSAIDs. Thus, without adequate controls, the relevance of these reports, though numerous, is in doubt; such cases may merely represent an aspect of the underlying disease process (Doherty et al., 1983).

This issue remains unresolved. Although two case-controlled retrospective studies have demonstrated apparent accelerated radiographic hip destruction in patients receiving NSAIDs (Ronningen and Langeland, 1979; Newman and Ling, 1985), a two-year prospective, placebo-controlled study of 89 patients with knee OA has failed to demonstrate increased radiological progression in those taking diclofenac (Dieppe et al., 1990). The numbers of patients involved in all these studies is, however, small and the possibility of a type II statistical error is high.

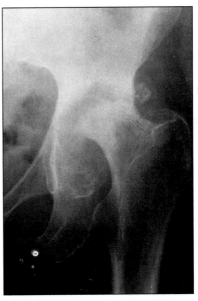

10.17

10.17 An example of 'Indocid hip' in a 72-year-old woman who has never received non-steroidal anti-inflammatory drugs.

10.18

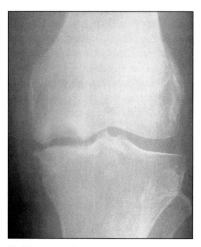

10.18 Avascular necrosis in a patient receiving systemic corticosteroids for asthma.

Steroids and joints

Corticosteroids either given systemically or intra-articularly have also been suggested to cause joint damage. There are many case reports in the literature of avascular necrosis in patients receiving systemic corticosteroid therapy (**10.18**). What is less clear, however, is whether less dramatic effects on joint metabolism can be produced which would result in a detrimental effect on the OA process. Work on animals, as already discussed, has even suggested a potentially chondroprotective effect of corticosteroids.

Many case reports have also described rapid joint destruction in association with intra-articular, particularly repeated, steroid injections. Large series of patients receiving repeated steroid injections have consistently failed to find a markedly increased risk of such destructive arthropathy (Gray *et al.*, 1981). Proper controlled studies in humans are, however, lacking.

Does chondroprotection exist in patients?

In spite of the difficulties, a number of putative CPAs have been tested in humans. However, for the most part, only symptomatic benefit, rather than chondroprotection has been demonstrated.

Azapropazone

A study comparing the rate of loss of cartilage and the time to operation of patients maintained on indomethacin or azapropazone, demonstrated an apparently better outcome in terms of time to hip replacement and decreased rate of joint space loss in those on azapropazone (Rashad *et al.*, 1989). This study is, however, readily criticised.

- The study was not blinded to the most important outcome measure, timing of surgery.
- The precise criteria for deciding the timing of surgery are not made explicit. Indeed, patients on indomethacin apparently had more effective pain relief, which may be a more important outcome measure, particularly in such a group of patients who all ultimately underwent surgery.
- The method of radiographic assessment, as discussed above, is imprecise. Indeed, many patients in both groups had an apparent increase in joint space.
- Statistical differences in the rate of joint space loss are apparent only on sub-group analysis. Patients who had apparent joint space increase were excluded.
- Biochemical differences were analysed only in a sub-group, the selection of which is not made clear.

The case for azapropazone as a CPA is unproven.

Tiaprofenic acid (TA)

Although much *in vitro* and animal work suggests TA is chondroprotective, human data are lacking. Two small studies demonstrate theoretically beneficial effects of TA on proteoglycans (Reginister *et al.*, 1985) and stromelysin (Vignon *et al.*, 1990). The clinical relevance of these observations is unclear.

Diclofenac

Although designed as a feasibility study of placebo-controlled trials in OA, no increase in the rate of radiographic progression was seen in patients treated with diclofenac slow-release 100 mg (Dieppe *et al.*, 1990), compared to those on placebo. However, only 51 of the 89 patients completed two years of therapy, with withdrawals mainly resulting from toxicity (5 placebo: 6 diclofenac) or lack of efficacy (3 diclofenac: 12 placebo).

Aspirin

Aspirin has been demonstrated to prevent cartilage degeneration in patients with recurrent patellar dislocation (Chrisman *et al.*, 1972). The relevance of such an effect to OA is unclear.

Glycosaminoglycans polysulphate (GAG-PS)

The use of this agent has been reviewed (Rejholec, 1987). Most studies exploring its use in patients have been open or uncontrolled, but there have also been placebo-controlled, double-blind studies. All these studies were relatively short-term: the longest was one year and although most demonstrated symptomatic efficacy for GAG-PS, none provide evidence of chondroprotection.

One long-term (5-year), single-blind placebo-controlled study has suggested both symptomatic improvement and more importantly a slowing of joint destruction in patients treated with GAG-PS (Rejholec, 1987).

Glycosaminoglycan-peptide complex (GP-C)

The use of this intramuscular agent in humans, has been reviewed (Rejholec, 1987). Again, although symptomatic benefit has been demonstrated, only two studies have provided evidence of chondroprotective effect.

A long-term (13-year) study of GP-C in patients with hip OA demonstrated both symptomatic benefit and a slowing of radiographic progression (Rejholec, 1987). Similar results were obtained in a 5-year, placebo-controlled single-blind study of knee and hip OA patients (Rejholec, 1987). Both GAG-PS and GP-C would appear to have chondroprotective action in humans but further confirmation is required.

Hyaluronic acid

Hyaluronic acid has been suggested to be a CPA but although it may produce symptomatic relief in double-blind, placebo-controlled studies, no evidence of a chondroprotective effect in humans has been demonstrated.

Orgotein

Although several studies have demonstrated good symptomatic responses to orgotein, none has yet demonstrated any chondroprotective effect.

Non-drug arthroprotection

Though study has mainly been concentrated on cartilage and bone abnormality, other joint tissues and other factors are also crucial in determining successful joint function. Usage has been well demonstrated to be necessary for satisfactory joint function; improvement in symptoms, function and well-being can be achieved with therapeutic exercise (Semble, 1990). Alteration of the biomechanics of the joint, for example by osteotomy, or the use of lateral insoles, or decreased impact on the joint, for example by improving muscle protective mechanisms or weight reduction, might enable the OA process to be successful, resulting in a 'compensated', asymptomatic outcome.

Chondroprotection at present

There is little convincing evidence that currently available drugs have a chondroprotective effect in patients. In spite of this, some agents are being marketed with claims to this effect. Such claims may be at best premature and at worst misplaced. Long-term prospective studies are still required to substantiate chondroprotection in humans. There may, however, be other reasons to avoid the use of potentially chondrodestructive drugs in OA. Indeed, there may be a current over-emphasis on the use of NSAIDs rather than simple analgesics for OA (Bradley et al., 1991). However, at present, avoidance of NSAIDs should be because of their side-effect profile and relative inefficacy, rather than consideration of any chondrodestructive or chondroprotective effects.

Chondroprotection in the future

In future, CPAs may be vitally important drugs, providing for the first time the ability to intervene directly in the OA process. Although in vitro and animal studies provide useful information, only long-term studies of large numbers of patients will determine whether chondroprotection is a valid concept in humans. Nevertheless, study of these drugs has helped provide evidence of the dynamic nature of the OA process and stimulated interest in the underlying pathophysiological mechanisms.

References and further reading

Bradley, J.D., Brandt, K.D., Katz, B.P., Kalasinski, L.A., Ryan, S.I. (1991) Comparison of an anti-inflammatory dose of ibuprofen, an analgesic dose of ibuprofen and acetaminophen in the treatment of patients with osteoarthritis of the knee. *New Eng. J. Med.*, **325**, 87–91.

Brandt, K.D. (1989) A pessimistic view of serologic markers for diagnosis and management of osteoarthritis. Biochemical, immunologic and clinicopathologic barriers. *J. Rheumatol.*, **16**, (Suppl 18), 39–42.

Burkhardt, D., Ghosh, P. (1987) Laboratory evaluation of antiarthritic drugs as potential chondroprotective agents. *Sem. Arthritis Rheum.*, **17** (Suppl 1), 3–34.

Chrisman, O.D., Snook, G.A., Wilson, T.C. (1972) The protective effect of aspirin against degeneration of human articular cartilage. *Clin. Orthop. Rel. Res.*, **84**, 193–196.

Coke, H. (1967) Long-term indomethacin treatment for coxarthrosis. *Ann. Rheum. Dis.*, **26**, 346–347.

Dieppe, P. (1990) Some recent clinical approaches to osteoarthritis research. *Sem. Arthritis Rheum.*, **20** (Suppl 1), 2–11.

Dieppe, P., Cushnaghan, J., Jasani, K., McCrae, F., Watt, I. (1993) A two-year placebo-controlled trial of a non-steroidal anti-inflammatory in therapy of the osteoarthritis of the knee joint. *Br. J. Rheumatol.*, **32** 595–600.

Doherty, M. (1989) 'Chondroprotection' by non-steroidal anti-inflammatory drugs. *Ann. Rheum. Dis.*, **48**, 619–621.

Doherty, M., Watt, I., Dieppe, P.A. (1983) Influence of primary generalised osteoarthritis on the development of secondary osteoarthritis. *Lancet*, **ii**, 8–11.

Doherty, M., Holt, M., MacMillan, P., Watt, L., Dieppe, P. (1986) A reappraisal of 'analgesic hip'. *Ann. Rheum. Dis.*, **45**, 272–276.

Gray, R.G., Tenenbaum, J., Gottlieb, N.L. (1981) Local corticosteroid injection treatment in rheumatic disorders. *Sem. Arthritis Rheum.*, **10**, 231–254.

Hutton, C.W., Higgs, E.R., Jackson, P.C., Watt, I. Dieppe, P.A., (1986) $^{99m}T_c$ HMDP bone scanning in generalized modal osteoarthritis. II. The four hour bone scan image predicts radiographic change. *Ann. Rheum. Dis.*, **45**, 622–626.

Kellgren, J.H., Lawrence, J.S. (1957) Radiological assessment of osteoarthritis. *Ann. Rheum. Dis.*, **16**, 494–502.

Newman, N.M., Ling, R.S.M. (1985) Acetabular bone destruction related to non-steroidal anti-inflammatory drugs. *Lancet*, **ii**, 11–14.

Pond, M.J., Nuki, G. (1973) Experimentally0induced osteoarthritis in the dog. *Ann. Rheum. Dis.*, **32**, 387–388.

Rashad, S., Revell, P., Hemingway, A., Low, F., Rainsford, K., Walker, F. (1989) Effect of non-steroidal anti-inflammatory drugs on the course of osteoarthritis. *Lancet*, **ii**, 519–522.

Reginister, J.Y., Gysen, P., Malaise, M., Franchimont, P. (1985) Influence of tiaprofenic acid on the synthesis and the physicochemical properties of articular proteoglycans in degenerative osteoarthritis and rheumatoid arthritis. In *New Trends in Rheumatology 3*, Nilsen, O.G. (Ed.), 53–58. Amsterdam: Excepta Medica SA.

Rejholec, V. (1987) Long-term studies of anti-osteoarthritic drugs: an assessment. *Sem. Arthritis Rheum.*, **17** (Suppl. 1), 35–53.

Ritter, M.A., Gioe, T.J. (1982) The effect of indomethacin on para-articular ectopic ossification following total hip arthroplasty. *Clin. Orthop.*, **167**, 113–117.

Ronningen, H., Langeland, N. (1979) Indomethacin treatment in osteoarthritis of the hip joint. *Acta Orthop. Scand.*, **50**, 169–174.

Semble, E.L., Loeser, R.F., Wise, C.M. (1990) Therapeutic exercise for rheumatoid arthritis and osteoarthritis. *Sem. Arthritis Rheum.*, **20**, 32–40.

Troyer, H. (1982) Experimental models of osteoarthritis: a review. *Sem. Arthritis Rheum.*, **11**, 362–374.

Vignon, E., Mathieu, P., Couprie, N., Cloppet, H., Herbage, D., Louisot, P., Richard, M. (1990) Effects of tiaprofenic acid on interleukin 1, phospholipase A2, neutral protease, and collagenase activity in rheumatoid synovial fluid. *Sem. Arthritis Rheum.*, **18** (Suppl 1), 11–15.

11. Surgical Treatment of Osteoarthritis

Ian Leslie

In the surgical management of osteoarthritis (OA) the prime aim is the relief of pain and in most patients this results in improvement of function. In some joints, function may not be restored unless movement is improved, e.g. the elbow joint, or stability improved, e.g. the knee joint. Unless these aims can be partially or wholly met, the value of the surgical procedure must be questioned.

Generally the surgeon is seeing the osteoarthritic joint at the end stage of its degenerative process and usually other conservative measures have failed, e.g. physiotherapy and drug treatment. Surgery is thus regarded by many as the salvage procedure to be sought when the patient has little or no alternative left. However, surgery also has a place in the prevention and perhaps the 'arrest' of OA.

This chapter, and of course much of the literature, addresses the surgical salvage of the degenerate joint, not by restoring the joint to normality but by providing a compromise for which the relief of pain and return of some function need to be traded off against the risks of surgical intervention, the longevity of the surgical procedure and subsequent salvage if that surgical procedure fails. Some procedures have been overtaken by the advancement of other techniques, such as total joint replacement. However, it is important to describe the older techniques in order to give an overview of the surgeon's attempts to relieve the pain and suffering associated with OA and also because some, if not all, still have a part to play. Total joint replacement is certainly not the only surgical operation for arthritis.

Prevention is better than cure and whilst most of the surgeon's work is involved in the salvage and removal of arthritic joints, surgery has a very definite part to play in the prevention of this condition.

Prevention

The surgeon's contribution to the prevention of OA lies mainly in the field of trauma. Direct damage to articular cartilage occurs at the moment of injury and this is an irreparable situation. The trauma may not only fracture the articular cartilage but may also fracture and displace the underlying foundation material, i.e. the subchondral bone. If part of the articular surface is displaced then this disrupts the intricate surface contact area between joints. Since load is then distributed over a smaller surface area then high pressure points result and the articular cartilage may not be able to withstand the subsequent pressures which will be exerted over the ensuing years. A depressed fracture of the tibial plateau may result in only 50% or less of the articular surface of the tibial plateau being available for articulation with the intact femoral condyle (**11.1, 11.2**). It is possible that the articular cartilage in most individuals would not stand such a high point loading for any length of time

without undergoing degenerative change. The surgeon can elevate the depressed articular cartilage of the tibial plateau, increase the strength of the foundations by inserting bone grafts beneath this area, and then maintain its position with modern techniques of internal fixation. Whilst the actual damage done to the articular cartilage is not repaired, the load distribution on this damaged cartilage is more evenly distributed and the articular cartilage is less likely to fail.

11.1   **11.2**

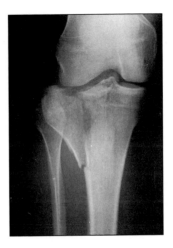 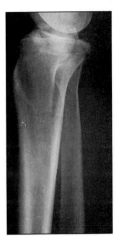

11.1, 11.2 The articular surface of the upper tibia has been completely disrupted by this tibial plateau fracture. The articular cartilage has been irreversibly damaged and the degenerative change would be aggravated by the incongruity of the articulation between the distal femur and the upper tibia. Surgical reconstruction can restore the congruity and allow early continuous passive mobilisation and thus minimise the risk of later degenerative change.

Even if the articular cartilage is not fractured and displaced, alteration in the position of the two articulating surfaces can also influence the congruity. This is best seen in the ankle joint where a 2mm displacement laterally will significantly alter the contoured arrangement of the articular surface of the tibia and the talus, producing areas of high load whilst off-loading other areas. The accuracy of reduction of these fracture-dislocations is an important factor in preventing the development of OA (**11.3**). Inaccurate reduction leads to degeneration (Burwell and Charnley, 1965). Modern methods of internal fixation allow accurate stable fixation and the possibility of early mobilisation (**11.4–11.7**).

11.3

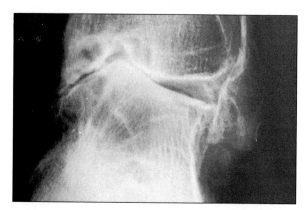

11.3 This fracture of the medial malleolus has been treated conservatively and has obviously displaced and healed in an abnormal position. The talus has tilted medially, mechnical forces have been concentrated on this side, and degenerative changes are inevitable. Fusion of this joint is the surgical option of choice.

11.4

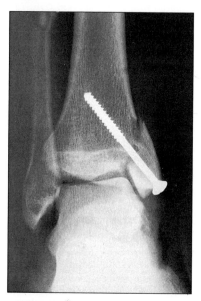

11.5

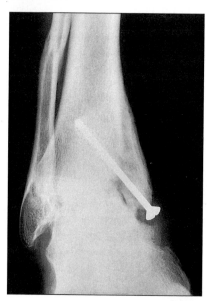

11.4, 11.5 There is a fracture of the medial malleolus (**11.4**) but the whole ankle mortice has been affected, as evidenced by the fracture of the fibula seen at the top of the picture. An attempt has been made to reduce and internally fix this fracture with one screw, but it can be seen that the fragment has not been accurately reduced. One year later (**11.5**), both fractures have united but there is a medial tilt on the talus and degenerative OA will be the result. Internal fixation alone does not restore the ankle to its normal position. Great care must be taken anatomically to reduce the fragments if degenerative change is to be avoided.

11.6

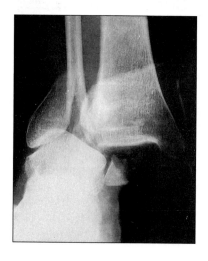

11.7

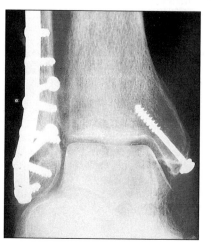

11.6, 11.7 A severe fracture dislocation of the ankle joint (**11.6**) involving both the medial and lateral malleoli. **11.7** shows the joint after modern methods of rigid internal fixation have been used. The reduction has been anatomical. The talus now lies in its normal position and at one year there is no evidence of any degenerative change. The prognosis for this ankle is excellent.

Instability is the result of ligamentous disruption or malalignment of the bones adjacent to the joint and may lead to excess shear forces being applied to the articular cartilage. This is perhaps best seen in the wrist joint where the malalignment of a distal radial fracture, e.g. Colles' fracture, disrupts the functioning position of the wrist, which after many years develops an instability pattern where the lunate is dorsally flexed and a zig-zag pattern occurs on the lateral view of the wrist joint. This type of instability pattern leads to weakness of grip together with pain and degenerative changes which may require surgical salvage (**11.8**, **11.9**).

Significant instability may develop in the patello-femoral or tibio-femoral joints after ligamentous injury to the knee. Abnormal movement occurring as a result sets up sheer stresses with which the articular cartilage cannot cope. The early correction of significant instabilities in the knee may help prevent the onset of OA, however, the long-term results of these types of procedures have yet to be evaluated.

Avascular necrosis may occur as a result of trauma. The damage to the vascular supply probably occurs at the time of injury but early restoration of anatomical alignment may allow the restoration of normal blood flow to the bone. This phenomenon is perhaps best seen in dislocation of the hip joint where the incidence of avascular necrosis can be related to the time between injury and the relocation of the joint, i.e. the longer the hip is dislocated the greater the chance of permanent vascular damage to the femoral head (Epstein, 1974). Where a fracture through the bone interrupts the blood supply to another part of the bone, then early restoration of anatomical alignment and stabilisation of the fracture gives the best chance of early revascularisation. Fractures of the neck of the femur and talus may result in avascular necrosis. The treatment of choice in order to reduce the incidence of

11.8

11.9

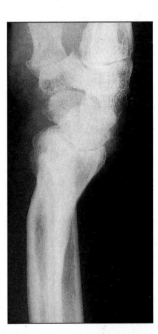

11.8, 11.9 This 56-year-old man suffered a fracture of his forearm at the age of 18 years. He worked in hard manual labour all his life and presented with symptoms of OA at the wrist joint. This fracture did not involve the articular surface but created a malalignment at the carpus, allowing the lunate to rotate dorsally and the capatate to rotate towards the palm. This creates a dorsal intercalated segmental instability which has led to the degenerative changes at the wrist joint. A fusion of the wrist was necessary to relieve the symptoms.

this avascularity is early reduction, open if necessary, and fixation of the fracture (**11.10–11.17**). This applies also to the carpal scaphoid fracture where significant displacement is best treated by early reduction and internal fixation.

When articular cartilage has been damaged then early motion appears to give it the greatest chance of survival. This has been well demonstrated in rabbits and this theory is now applied to articular injury in humans. The long period of immobilisation of joint injuries which has been practised in the past, has been superseded by the process of early continuous passive mobilisation. Obviously, this requires stability of the joint, which can be achieved by various methods of

11.10

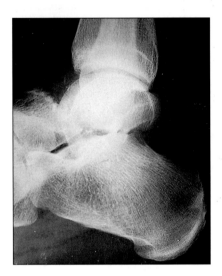

11.11

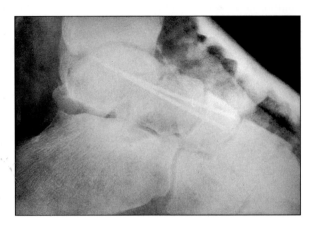

11.10, 11.11 A displaced fracture of the neck of the talus (**11.10**). The blood supply to the body of the talus is in jeopardy. In **11.11** the fracture has been reduced within six hours and internally fixed with two Kirschner wires. Early reduction and maintenance of that reduction by internal fixation reduces the chance of avascular necrosis of the talus with subsequent collapse and degenerative change within the ankle joint.

11.12   **11.13**   **11.14**

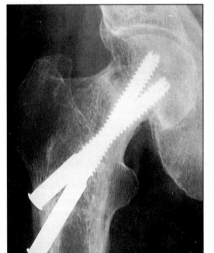

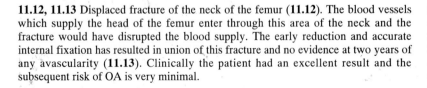

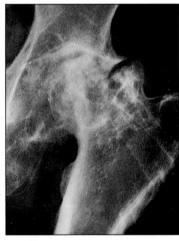

11.14 This patient had a similar displaced fracture of the neck of the femur to that shown in **11.12**. Despite adequate reduction and internal fixation the superior segment of the femoral head has undergone necrosis and collapse with subsequent degenerative changes necessitating total hip replacement.

11.12, 11.13 Displaced fracture of the neck of the femur (**11.12**). The blood vessels which supply the head of the femur enter through this area of the neck and the fracture would have disrupted the blood supply. The early reduction and accurate internal fixation has resulted in union of this fracture and no evidence at two years of any avascularity (**11.13**). Clinically the patient had an excellent result and the subsequent risk of OA is very minimal.

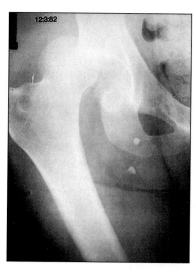
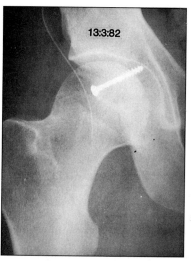
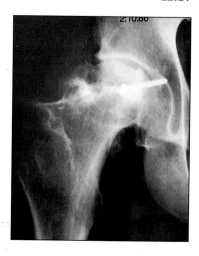

11.15–11.17 This patient suffered a fracture-dislocation of the hip in a road traffic accident (**11.15**). The hip joint has been opened and reduced (**11.16**) and a fragment of bone in the posterior wall of the acetabulum has been fixed in place. Despite the early operation and reduction, the superior segment of the femoral head has undergone necrosis and degenerative change (**11.17**). These changes are often slow to appear but usually become evident during the subsequent two years. This young patient could be treated by an arthrodesis or total hip replacement.

internal fixation, and then immediately postoperatively the limb is placed on a machine which moves the joint through a set range of motion on a continuous basis for as long as is practicable. There is no doubt that this leads to a much earlier return of joint function and seemingly to an early reduction in pain. The long-term effects of continuous passive mobilisation have yet to be evaluated but so far it does seem extremely helpful in the prevention of degenerative changes. For the trauma surgeon the aim of surgical treatment of joint injuries is the early restoration of joint movement and the return of muscle function. These principles would appear to bode well for the long-term future of the injured joint.

The aim of surgical treatment of childhood conditions is not only to improve the function of the joint, but also to prevent later degeneration (**11.18**). This is best seen in the treatment of Perthes' disease where, after a short irritable phase, the child is asymptomatic yet may undergo a surgical intervention in order to reduce the chance of the development of OA during adult life. Slipped upper femoral epiphysis will lead to joint malalignment and early OA. Surgical stabilisation of a slipping epiphysis will reduce the chance of a malformed femoral head with its subsequent degenerative problems.

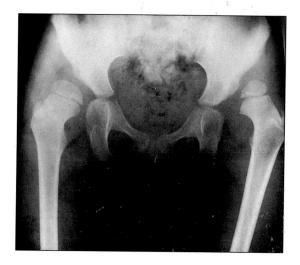

11.18 Congenital dislocation of the left hip with acetabular dysplasia of the right hip which allows the femoral head to sublux laterally. Both hip joints in this patient will undergo degenerative changes during early adult life. The early diagnosis of this condition is essential for the prevention of OA. In view of the totally dislocated hip on the left side the patient will also have a very ugly gait.

Surgical treatment of the OA joint

Physicians and surgeons have, for many years, been trying to relieve the pain of arthritic joints. It would seem that the only permanent way of surgically treating the arthritic joint is to remove it. This can be achieved by:

- Eliminating the joint altogether and joining the two bones across that area, i.e. an arthrodesis.
- Removing the joint and leaving an empty space producing a pseudoarthrosis.
- Removing the joint and replacing one or both sides of the joint.

Each of these salvage procedures has its own advantages and disadvantages. None will restore the joint to its natural state, i.e. pain-free, with a full range of motion and lasting 90 to 100 years. Since the aim of surgical treatment is the elimination of pain, then it would be helpful if the origin of the pain was accurately known. Unfortunately this is not the case. However, many operations have been devised to eliminate pain from the joint without eliminating the joint itself and these will be dealt with first before the procedures which eliminate the joint altogether are described.

Neurectomy

The sensation of pain arising from a joint reaches the central nervous system mainly via the peripheral nerves and a logical step in the reduction of this pain is to obliterate this input. This can be achieved by dividing the peripheral nerves which supply a joint. The concern about doing a neurectomy is that it may produce a Charcot-type joint. However, it has become apparent that it is impossible to obliterate all sensation from a joint by merely sectioning the peripheral nerves. Some of the sensory input travels with the blood vessels and it is only by surgical section of the spinal cord, where these nerves are conjoined, that total ablation can be achieved. The proponents of neurectomy never found that a Charcot-type arthropathy resulted from peripheral denervation (Bateman, 1948). The pattern of innervation of a joint is an anatomical limiting factor for surgical denervation. The knee, hip and elbow have well-defined and distinct articular branches which can be identified with some degree of consistency, whereas the shoulder, wrist and ankle have a much greater scatter of nerves and therefore it is more difficult to achieve denervation (Casagrande *et al.*, 1951).

Most interest has centred round denervation of the hip joint where the major branches arrive via the obturator, sciatic and femoral nerves. These three nerves must be exposed for a satisfactory result. The obturator nerve is perhaps the most important to divide, but to get reasonable pain relief then branches of all three must be cut (Kaplan, 1948; Mulder 1948).

At the elbow joint the median and ulnar nerves as well as the posterior interosseous and radial nerves must be exposed and branches divided (Bateman, 1948).

Generally, neurectomy has gone out of fashion for the treatment of the osteoarthritic joint. However, one operation still remains in vogue for the treatment of wrist pain, and that is the division of the posterior interosseous nerve of the forearm as it crosses the distal end of the radius.

Muscle decompression

The hip joint has been a constant area of interest in OA. A method of relieving the pain was advocated by O'Malley (1959), in which the tendons of the psoas muscle and the adductors of the hip joint were divided and an anterior capsulotomy performed. He described 200 cases in which 85% had a complete, or near complete, loss of pain. Whilst this operation was practised by many it has not gained universal acceptance and is probably not performed any more.

Bone decompression

It has been postulated that the source of pain, especially pain at rest, is venous congestion within the subchondral bone. The success of osteotomy has been attributed to the relief of this pressure and the change in the subchondral circulation (Helal, 1965). Therefore a logical step forward in order to relieve pain is to decompress the intramedullary bone and allow improved venous drainage. This method has been used with variable success. In 1936 MacKenzie reported on 106 femoral drillings and 80% of his patients had good relief of pain. However, the follow-up period was not specified. In a presentation to the Royal Society of Medicine in 1956, Agerholn-Christensen and Gleave stated that they had performed 125 such operations and reported on 30 of these, 50% of whom had good relief of pain. However, Leach in 1963 passed a Steinman pin from the lateral cortex of the femur up the femoral neck and then drilled a 12 mm hole to within 12 mm of the subchondral bone. Ten operations were performed on nine patients. All had good relief of pain which lasted for six months in six patients, but a shorter period of time in the others. At follow-up, at two years, only one had a good result and one had a fair result. He therefore abandoned this procedure. Generally, cortical drilling has lost favour, although some surgeons will drill the femoral cortex just below the tip of a hip joint prosthesis in order to relieve nonspecific femoral pain after hip replacement.

Core decompression may well have a place in the treatment of avascular necrosis of bone. Solomon (1981) stated that a 7 mm core taken out of the femoral neck probably alters the progression of ischaemic necrosis in Stage I and probably also in Stage II. Zizic and Hungerford (1985) reported on 211 patients who had core decompression for osteonecrosis of bone. Further surgery was required only in 4% of those who had a Stage I disease at the time of decompression and in 23% of those who had Stage II osteonecrosis. It is thought that the improvement occurs because of the venous decompression that takes place and is based on the assumption that ischaemic necrosis of bone is not necessarily just caused by lack of input of blood but also by lack of outflow producing stagnant ischaemia. Whilst bone decompression would not appear to be of any value in the treatment of OA of the hip it would seem to have a place in the prevention of progression of ischaemic necrosis of bone which, of course, leads to OA (Zizic and Hungerford, 1985).

Joint debridement

Magnuson in 1946 described joint debridement as being of value in the treatment of pain in the osteoarthritic knees in overweight women past the age of 40 years. It was indicated in the less severely involved knee and the joint was exposed much as it is nowadays for a total knee replacement. An osteotome was used to remove the osteophytes from both condyles, the degenerated cartilage was shaved from the condyles down to cancellous bone, and the patella was narrowed. The semilunar cartilages were left in place unless they were damaged. Hyaluronidase was then instilled into the joint. It is stated that 60 out of 62 patients were relieved of their symptoms following this procedure.

Pridie in 1959 described the drilling of the areas of exposed bone within a degenerative knee joint (**11.19–11.21**). After the debridement, multiple drill holes were made to encourage a blood supply which would regenerate in those situations but mainly as a fibrocartilage and not as an articular cartilage.

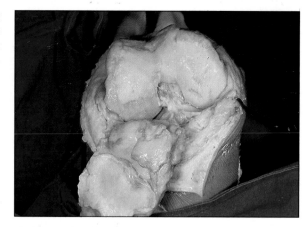

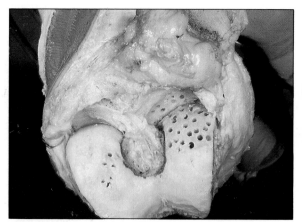

11.20

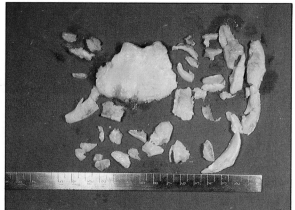

11.19–11.21 Gross degenerative arthritis is shown in this knee joint (**11.19**). The articular cartilage on the femoral condyle has been worn away down to the subchondral bone (eburnation) and there are multiple osteophytes around the rim of the femoral condyle as well as the patella. In **11.20** a 'Pridie' operation has been performed. The osteophytes and menisci have been removed and multiple drill holes have been made in areas of articular cartilage loss. **11.21** shows the debris that has been removed during the debridement of the knee joint. Note that the whole articular surface of the patella has been removed and subchondral bone is exposed.

Insall (1974) followed up 62 of Pridie's patients for two-and-a-half years and found that 77% considered that they had a good result. Whilst this procedure is not now used for widespread OA of joints, many surgeons still drill small areas of cartilage loss in order to stimulate fibrocartilage formation. Recent attempts to stimulate the healing of articular cartilage defects have involved the filling of the defect with a pad of woven carbon fibre. Significant pain relief has been reported in over 70% of patients. The open weave appears to facilitate the ingrowth of fibrous tissue (Muckle and Minns, 1990).

Cheilectomy has formed part of the surgical procedure of debridement of the joint for OA. However, it can be used in isolation in certain instances where osteophyte formation is painfully obstructing joint motion. This is perhaps most commonly encountered in the elbow joint and the first metatarsophalangeal joint, where it is seen in the form of hallux rigidus.

Joint lavage and abrasion arthroplasty

With the increased use of the arthroscope for the diagnosis and surgical treatment of conditions of the knee joint, it was noted that many patients gained relief of osteoarthritic symptoms following a diagnostic arthroscopy. During this procedure, saline or Hartmann's solution is used to irrigate the joint and in so doing removes the debris which may be acting as a synovial irritant. Therefore, joint lavage has become popular as a method of treating OA of the knee joint, particularly in those cases which have an inflammatory component such as crystal arthropathy. With the introduction of powered tools, debridement can also be carried out using arthroscopic techniques (Johnson, 1986). A protected power-burr is inserted into the knee and the osteophytes and loose cartilage fragments removed. At the same time the exposed subchondral bone can be abraded producing a bleeding surface in the hopes of stimulating fibrocartilage formation. However, abrasion arthroplasty and debridement would not appear to be permanent solutions to the osteoarthritic knee. Rogan (1989) has performed these procedures on 49 patients who had prolonged symptoms with recent exacerbations not resolving on conservative treatment. At follow-up between 12 and 24 months later, 20 had an excellent result, 12 were good, 11 were the same and two were worse. However, it appears that two to four years after the procedure problems recur and it could perhaps be regarded as a method which produces relief of pain and could be seen as delaying the necessity for joint replacement.

Schonholtz (1989) considers that arthroscopic debridement is a valuable alternative to joint replacement. It is palliative in nature and can yield permanent relief in the low-demand knee of the elderly patient. He thought the procedure was also valuable in the young knee which was not yet ready for reconstruction. The risk/benefit ratio was considered favourable.

Osteotomy

Osteotomy, or division of the bone adjacent to the joint, remains an option in modern surgery. The reason for the success of the osteotomy is controversial, but it is clear that several things are achieved:

* The arterial and, more particularly, the venous circulation are altered. This relieves the venous congestion and by that method alone may relieve the rest pain (Anoldi, 1975).
* The mechanical forces acting across the joint can be deliberately altered, and the realignment of the axis of weight-bearing can take the pressure off one area of the joint and distribute it more evenly over the entire joint. This is seen particularly in upper tibial osteotomy for the correction of genu varum (bow leg) deformity associated with OA of the medial tibiofemoral compartment.
* The joint position can be altered so that an area of the joint which still has articular cartilage can be brought into the weight-bearing position, and the area which has lost its articular cartilage can be taken away from that position to be put into an area of minimal weight-bearing. This is possible in joints which have a large surface area of which only part is taking the full load in the normal standing position. The hip joint lends itself to this type of operation because it has the potential for multiplanar alterations of position. By taking radiographs in various positions of abduction, adduction, flexion and rotation, a position is sought where the weight-bearing joint space is increased on the radiograph and then a sub-trochanteric osteotomy is performed so that the head is maintained in that position, whilst the remainder of the limb is brought back to the neutral position.
* There is relief of tension in the surrounding tissue, particularly the capsule and adjacent muscles.

Osteotomy should not be considered a cure for OA. Nissen (1963) described it as an 'arrest of OA'.

A popular form of osteotomy in the region of the hip joint was the McMurray displacement osteotomy. No attention was paid to planning a geometrical osteotomy. The bone was divided and the shaft displaced medially and allowed to heal. This produced extremely good results in terms of pain relief and in many patients a regeneration of a joint space was seen (**11.22, 11.23**). This type of osteotomy is hardly ever performed now. The shaft of the femur is offset and negotiation of the femoral canal with a straight metal stem of a subsequent hip prosthesis causes difficulties.

A dorsal wedge osteotomy of the proximal phalanx of the great toe is useful in the treatment of hallux rigidus as it places the articular surface of the phalanx in a more plantar-flexed resting position (Citron and Neil, 1987). Osteotomy of the first metacarpal is also recommended for the symptomatic OA of the trapeziometacarpal joint of the thumb.

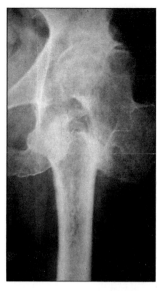
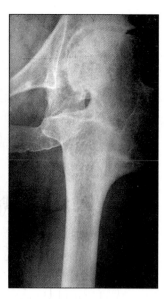

11.22, 11.23 A McMurray's osteotomy has been performed for OA of the hip (**11.22**). The shaft of the femur has been displaced medially and the bone allowed to heal in that new position without any internal fixation. **11.23** shows the same hip five years later and there is now restoration of the joint space.

Elimination of the joint

The permanent surgical solution to OA is to eliminate the joint. It may be excised and the ends of the two adjacent bones may be put together to form a single bone (arthrodesis) or else the joint may be totally excised and the gap between them filled with material which allows painless motion. This material may be the patient's own tissue, i.e. a pseudoarthrosis or a facial interposition arthroplasty. It may be filled with a plastic or metal material, e.g. silastic or titanium. The gap may be filled by a structure which has an articulating facility similar to the original joint, i.e. replacement arthroplasty.

Arthrodesis

Any joint may be arthrodesed, although some are a little more difficult to fuse than others. Whilst a successful arthrodesis will relieve pain and will confer upon the joint absolute stability, it is at the price of loss of movement. In some joints this is not of a significant functional disadvantage. For example an arthrodesis of two vertebrae within the lumbar spine does not reduce the movement in the spine sufficiently to confer any functional disability. An arthrodesis of the first metatarsophalangeal joint in the foot improves pain and the lack of movement does not cause a significant problem, unless the position of the arthrodesis is incorrect. Likewise, the ankle joint and the wrist joint can be arthrodesed with minimal functional loss.

However, an arthrodesed knee, hip or elbow will cause significant disadvantages. In order to compensate for the loss of movement at one joint, those above or below that particular joint should have a good range of motion. If not, these adjacent joints cannot compensate for the loss of movement. For example, fusion of the carpometacarpal joint of the thumb will not be successful if the scaphotrapezial joint also has OA and pain restricts its movement. An arthrodesis of both knees or hip joints will cause considerable mobility problems, especially for climbing stairs, sitting down and rising from the floor after falling down.

Where stability is the essence, then arthrodesis is very satisfactory. However, where mobility is required then arthrodesis is unsatisfactory and an alternative method of joint pain relief must be sought.

An arthrodesis may be intra-articular; intra- and extra-articular; or extra-articular. The choice of technique for any given case will depend upon the age of the patient, the pathological process involving the joint and the presence or absence of gross deformity of the joint.

With an intra-articular arthrodesis the articular surfaces are denuded of all remaining cartilage as well as the subchondral sclerotic bone, so that the two cancellous areas of bone may be approximated (**11.24**). These two bones must then be rigidly stabilised otherwise any movement occurring will produce a pseudoarthrosis which may well then be painful. Compression of the two surfaces produces excellent stability and this enhances bone healing. Compression can be achieved by passing pins through the bone above and below the joint and applying an external clamp. This method was popularised by Sir John Charnley for arthrodesis of the knee and the ankle joint (**11.25, 11.26**). More sophisticated and somewhat more complex compression techniques are now available. Internal fixation in the form of plates and screws or pins passed across the joint eliminates the need for exposed pins (**11.27**). A successful method of achieving fusion of the knee joint after the excision of a failed arthroplasty is to pass a very long Kuntschner nail down through the femur, across the knee joint and into the tibia.

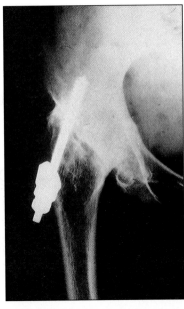

11.24

11.24 An arthrodesis of the hip has been performed using internal fixation.

11.25

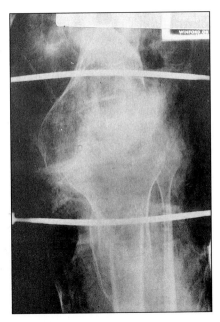

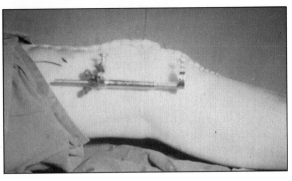

11.26

11.25, 11.26 This knee has been arthrodesed by resection of the end of the femur and the upper end of the tibia (**11.25**). The two surfaces are being compressed by external fixation. The forces being applied through the knee joint are demonstrated by the bend of the Steinman pins which pass through the lower femur and the upper tibia. A Charnley clamp is well-tolerated by the patient and a thumb-screw allows the compression to be increased with time (**11.26**). Rigid stability can be obtained by this compression method.

11.27

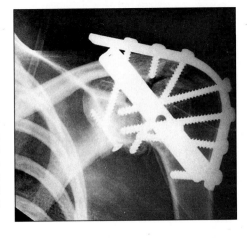

11.27 Rigid internal fixation may be used for arthrodesis of certain joints. Here a shoulder has been arthrodesed by two plates and multiple bone screws following the AO method. The advantage is that a plaster spica is not required and the mobility of the elbow and scapulothoracic area can be maintained. It may be necessary to remove these plates once the arthrodesis has consolidated.

11.28

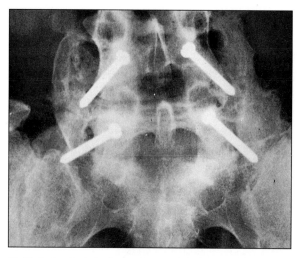

Extra-articular arthrodesis is achieved by placing cortical and corticocancellous bone across the outside of a joint with or without clearing the articular surfaces (**11.28**). This method is quite effective in joints which have been subject to infection where the surgeon may not wish to enter the joint, and where the articular surface has been grossly destroyed by the infective process. Many of these forms of arthrodesis do involve prolonged immobilisation which may be considered a distinct disadvantage, especially if it means lying in bed with a hip or shoulder spica. With the use of rigid internal fixation or compression external fixation, this disadvantage can be overcome.

11.28 Arthrodesis is the treatment of choice for OA of the spine. Here screw fixation is supplemented by bone graft between the transverse processes of L4, L5 and S1. Movement at these levels will be totally restricted and therefore increased movement and stress will occur at the intervertebral joints above this level. This may lead to accelerated degenerative changes higher up the spine.

Arthroplasty

Another way of eliminating the osteoarthritic joint is to replace it with something else so that movement is maintained between the two adjacent bones. An arthroplasty can be one of the following types:

- **Excision arthroplasty.** The joint surfaces are excised, and the bone ends deliberately kept apart, so that the resulting haematoma is eventually reorganised into a thick layer of fibrous scar tissue (**11.29**).
- **Interpositional arthroplasty.** The joint is excised and the bone ends kept apart by the insertion of a piece of the patient's own fascia or muscle, or a piece of man-made material such as silastic (**11.30**).
- **Replacement arthroplasty.** The joint is excised and replaced with a man-made device which is attached to the bone ends and mechanically tries to simulate the normal motion of the joint. The replacement may be of one side of the joint only (hemi-arthroplasty) or both surfaces (total arthroplasty).
- **Allograft arthroplasty.** The joint is excised and the joint from a donor is fixed in its place.

11.29

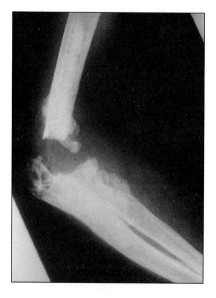

11.30

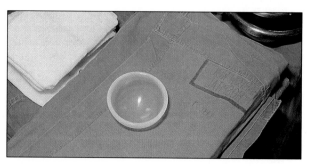

11.30 This silastic cup is used as an interposition arthroplasty and placed between the head of the humerus and the glenoid. It is used most often in the treatment of rheumatoid arthritis.

11.29 An excisional arthroplasty of the elbow has been performed. This allows excellent pain-free mobility but unfortunately instability is a problem. It is difficult to lift weights, e.g. to support a pot of tea.

<u>Excision arthroplasty</u> Whilst excision arthroplasty produces excellent relief of pain, it is necessary to sacrifice the stability of the joint. It is thus totally unsuitable for a knee joint or an intervertebral joint. In other joints some degree of stability can be maintained, e.g. the hip joint. Excision arthroplasty is quite successful for the following joints:

- **The acromioclavicular joint.** Excision of the outer 1.5 cm of the clavicle produces little functional disability and is often performed in association with an acromioplasty for rotator cuff impingement syndromes. The osteophytes on the under-surface of this joint may interfere with the function of the supraspinatus tendon and failure to deal with this problem may preclude a good result from that type of surgery.
- **Radial head excision.** Whilst this is most commonly performed for rheumatoid arthritis of the elbow joint, it is also quite successful in the management of comminuted fractures of the radial head and is of benefit for post-traumatic arthritis which may result from that. It allows full supination and pronation to be achieved, presuming the distal radio-ulnar joint is not involved. However, in the post-traumatic case, some proximal migration of the radius may occur with some disruption of the relationship at the distal radio-ulnar joint.
- **Excision of the distal end of the ulna.** This is most commonly performed for rheumatoid arthritis. However, degenerative change may occur at this joint as a result of malunion of a distal-radial fracture and excision of the distal 1 to 2 cm of this bone (Darrach's procedure) improves the rotational range of the forearm and reduces pain.
- **Proximal row carpectomy.** Stamm in 1944 described excision of the proximal row for the treatment of arthrosis of the carpus. This operation is still considered to be successful for secondary degenerative change resulting from non-union of the scaphoid, Keinbock's disease or traumatic instabilities of the carpus (Crabbe, 1964; Inglis and Jones, 1977). It offers good relief of pain and moderate stability whilst retaining wrist motion.
- **Metacarpophalangeal joints.** Kestler in 1946 described a procedure where the metacarpal head is excised, mainly in the treatment of rheumatoid arthritis. This resulted in some loss of extension of the MP joint but a gain of approximately 50° in flexion. When this operation is performed now a silastic prosthesis is usually inserted between the stump of the metacarpal and the proximal phalanx.
- **Carpometacarpal joint of the thumb.** Excision of the trapezium remains a popular operation for OA of the carpometacarpal joint of the thumb. Whilst it does not maintain the same pinch grip as would an arthrodesis, it preserves mobility and certainly improves the pain and therefore hand function. It is essential to excise the trapezium, rather than arthodese it, if there is also scaphotrapezial OA. Excellent long-term results can be achieved (Gervis, 1949; Murley, 1960).
- **Hip joint.** In 1945 Girdlestone recorded the results of excision arthroplasty of the hip in 25 patients. Fourteen of these were rated as excellent, 5 as good and 3 as poor. Other types of pseudoarthroses have been described and although pain is relieved and mobility restored, there is some significant disadvantage in the resulting shortening, and a degree of instability. Rock and Bourne (1981) reviewed patients who had a Girdlestone pseudoarthrosis and found that 90% had good relief of pain, although when it was performed as a primary procedure 90% were dissatisfied. When the operation had been performed as a secondary procedure, i.e. after some other type of surgery which had failed, then only 40% were dissatisfied. There was an average of 4.5 cm of shortening. When assessed objectively 18% of those who had a primary operation and 50% of those with a secondary operation were rated as fair to good. However, this operation remains a salvage procedure for those patients who have a grossly infected total hip replacement. McElwaine and Colville (1984) stated that 13 out of the 22 patients had no pain at all following the procedure but had a poor functional result with instability and fatigue, and need for support. The pain that they suffered from their infected hip replacement had been greatly improved (*see* **11.36**).
- **Patellofemoral joint.** Excision of the patella has been performed quite frequently for isolated patellofemoral arthritis. Approximately 75% of patients will have a good or fair result, with some resulting weakness in knee extension (Ackroyd and Polyzoides, 1978; French, 1959).
- **Metatarsophalangeal joint of the great toe.** This is perhaps the most frequently performed excisional arthroplasty and is generally termed a Keller's operation. The proximal half of the proximal phalanx of the great toe is excised and the exostosis removed. Many patients are extremely satisfied; however it does tend to defunction the great toe and may occasionally transfer weight laterally on to the other metatarsal heads where the patient may develop pain. The toe is shortened and slightly floppy, but is generally pain-free.

Interpositional arthroplasty Excision of the joint and placing between it a biologically compatible plastic or metal component achieves pain relief and allows movement. However, like excision arthroplasty, instability may be a problem.

The elbow joint, being an upper limb hinge joint, has lent itself to interpositional arthroplasty using fascia to cover the bone ends. Excellent results have been achieved, although instability still remains a problem. The introduction of metal as an interposing material is best seen in the use of the vitallium cups which were placed over the femoral head by Smith-Petersen as early as 1938. Cup-arthroplasty in the hip joint became a popular operation and early results were good, with up to 80% of cases being free from pain (Law, 1948). The operation required the complete removal of the synovium and of the articular surfaces down to cancellous bone. Postoperatively the patient was maintained on active movements whilst on traction, and was then allowed up with crutches at the end of five weeks. Full weight-bearing was not permitted for six months. However, problems associated with pressure atrophy on the acetabulum or the femoral head and neck, and the occurrence of new bone formation around the joint eventually limited its use.

Interpositional arthroplasty using fascia, and/or rolled up tendons, is still used in the treatment of carpometacarpal joint arthritis of the thumb, after trapeziectomy. The material most often used for interposition is a silastic polymer shaped like a trapezium. Occasionally silastic is used to replace the radial head and to cover the distal end of the ulna, after excision of the head (Darrach's procedure). Silastic sheeting may be used between joint surfaces and has been of some value in rheumatoid arthritis of the elbow and OA of the base of the thumb. Silastic sheet in the form of a cup has also been found useful in rheumatoid arthritis of the shoulder (*see* **11.30**). The concern with silastic has centred around the aggressive synovitis which may develop, probably as a result of the size of the silastic particles which are worn away by joints which are subject to shearing and compression forces (Carter *et al.*, 1986). This produces radiographic evidence of resorption and cyst formation in the bone adjacent to the silastic implant.

Replacement arthroplasty Replacement of a joint by metal, plastic or ceramics is now the most popular surgical method of treatment of OA. This concept is not new but advances in technology and an increased knowledge of the reaction of human tissue to implants has led to a major industrial expansion in this field. In 1922 Hey-Groves replaced the femoral head with an ivory prosthesis. Plastic materials were used by the Judet brothers in the 1940s. In the 1950s Thompson as well as Moore produced the metal femoral head, with a stem for the femoral shaft. Whilst these are not generally used for OA, they are in very wide use for the treatment of displaced fractures of the femoral neck in the elderly. In the early 1960s the replacement of the femoral head with a metal ball and stem, and the replacement of the acetabulum with a metal cup, was popularised by McKee and Watson-Farrar (**11.31**). This prosthesis gained immense popularity and relieved the pain and suffering of OA of the hip for many thousands of people. It was thought, however, that the metal-upon-metal prosthesis had a high friction coefficient and this produced torsional forces on the components resulting in early loosening. The late Sir John Charnley developed what he called a low-friction arthroplasty in which a metal head articulated with a plastic acetabular socket (Charnley, 1961; **11.32**). An early set-back in Charnley's work was his use of a teflon plastic cup. Whilst it had a low-friction coefficient, it also had poor wear qualities, but when he replaced this plastic component with high-density polyethylene, the success of this type of hip replacement was established. Except for some minor modifications to stem design, materials and cementing techniques, the Charnley prosthesis still enjoys an unprecedented popularity in the treatment of OA of the hip. The long-term results are excellent and it is still used as the standard against which all other types of hip prostheses are compared.

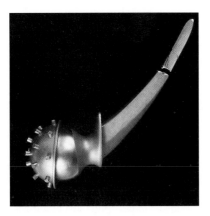

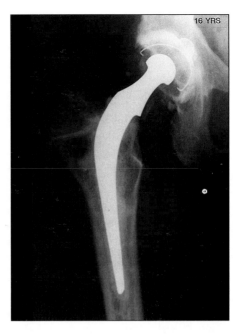

11.31 A McKee-Farrar total hip replacement. This is the forerunner of the present day total hip replacement and used a metal cup fixed to the acetabulum by acrylic cement. The spikes on the cup assisted in the fixation of the metal cup within the cement. A metal ball articulated with the metal cup and this was held by a stem which passed down the femur and was held there by acrylic cement. Metal fatigue was a problem and stress fractures did occur, as seen in this picture. Fractures of the stem are now very uncommon because of the improved metallurgical techniques.

11.32 This Charnley total hip replacement has been in place for 16 years and the patient remains totally asymptomatic. The radio-opaque methylmethacrylate cement can be seen in the acetabulum and surrounding the femoral component. The ghost shadows of screw holes are also seen in the femoral shaft. This patient had a previous osteotomy with an internal fixation device.

These three pioneers, McKee, Watson-Farrar and Charnley, also led in the development of the use of acrylic cement in bone as a method of fixing the prosthesis.

One of the problems in the use of total joint arthroplasty is the fixation of the metal or plastic prosthesis to living bone. The use of methyl-methacrylate cement has stood the test of time, although granulomatous reaction and subsequent bone resorption may develop around the cement-bone interface with associated loosening of the prosthesis and pain. A significant amount of bone stock can be lost, producing difficulties for insertion of another prosthesis.

Attention has been focused, therefore, on uncemented prosthesis. The surface of the prosthesis has been altered in many ways in order to stimulate the local bone to grow into and around the new prosthesis – so-called 'osseous integration'. Titanium has been successful, as has the coating of a prosthesis with hydroxy-apatite. Ceramics have also proved extremely popular, especially biocompatibility and wear, and these products do not appear to be reactive, as are those made of acrylic cement and metals.

The concerns with total joint replacement, particularly in young patients, are the longevity of the prosthesis and the ability to salvage a situation by replacement with another prosthesis. Unlike the patient with rheumatoid arthritis, the young patient with single major joint involvement with OA, who has a successful joint replacement, will resume his or her normal physical activity, and this places great stresses across the artificial joint and its interface with the living bone. Current research and development is thus orientated towards increased longevity by reducing wear at the articular surface and loosening at the bone interface. Attempts are also being made to produce a femoral component for the total hip replacement which has a coefficient of elasticity similar to that of bone.

Infection is the great enemy of total joint arthroplasty. Whether acute or of a low-grade nature, it causes bone resorption, death of surrounding bone, loosening of the prosthesis, pain and thus failure of the whole procedure. In the past such a complication would have meant the removal of the prosthesis and the formation of a pseudoarthrosis (**11.33–11.36**). The failed hip replacement can perform satisfactorily with a pseudoarthrosis, although patients are generally far from satisfied, even though their pain is relieved. (McElwaine and Colville, 1984). At the knee joint an arthrodesis has to be performed and this can be extremely difficult to achieve after removal of a prosthesis because of the large amount of bone that has already been removed and the presence of the infected tissue, which has also caused significant osteoporosis.

More recently, it has been possible to replace an infected prosthesis. Thorough debridement of all the granulomatous tissue and dead bone, the use of antibiotic-loaded cement, as well as systemic antibiotics, has resulted in a satisfactory salvage rate (Bucholz *et al.*, 1981).

Great efforts are always made to prevent infection during and after these operations. Operating theatres with laminar-flow of air to prevent turbulence and thus the deposit of bacteria-laden dust in the wound, the use of barriers which totally isolate the surgeon from the patient, the use of antibiotic-loaded cements and the peroperative use of systemic antibiotics, have all helped to reduce the infection rate to less than 1%.

In the hip joint, dislocation can be a persistent problem, even after 15 years, when, as a result of wear of the plastic cup, the shape of the acetabulum is altered and the prosthesis dislocates unexpectedly. This probably requires revision surgery.

Total arthroplasty of the knee joint has progressed rapidly over the past 10 years and a 60% to 70% success rate 10 years ago has improved greatly to come close to the success rate of hip replacements, i.e. around 94%. The many designs of knee joint replacement perhaps indicate how difficult it has been to overcome the mechanical problems. The long-term results of the more modern prostheses are not yet available, but it is to be hoped that they will match those of the Charnley hip replacement.

Whilst the hip joint was probably the easiest total arthroplasty problem to solve, followed by the knee joint, these are by no means the only successful ones. Other joints are being replaced and are perhaps still at the developmental stage which the knee joint was at 10 years ago. In particular, replacement of the elbow joint is now highly successful, especially in the rheumatoid patient, and is certainly of value in some patients with OA (**11.37, 11.38**). Total replacement of the shoulder joint is now gaining significantly better results. Total replacement of the wrist joint has been less successful because of the problem of bone–prosthesis fixation, and perhaps the most successful wrist joint prosthesis so far is the Swanson silastic hinge. This is not so much a total joint replacement but more an anatomical interpositional arthroplasty. Whilst replacement of the ankle joint is available, its results have to compete with the other extremely successful alternative, i.e. ankle arthrodesis.

An artificial joint can never match the natural joint, will not last as long, will not stand the stresses and will not have the same range of motion and the same degree of stability.

11.33

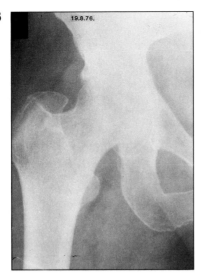

11.34

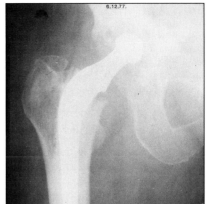

11.33–11.36 This lady has symptomatic OA of the right hip (**11.33**). A Charnley total hip replacement has been successfully performed but at 15 months there is some resorption of bone at the calcar of the femur (**11.34**). This patient developed a late deep-seated infection.

11.35

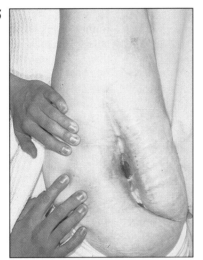

11.36

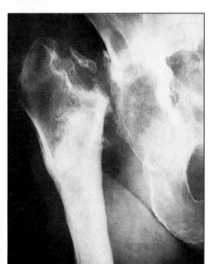

A chronic discharging wound is seen over the site of the hip replacement (**11.35**). In **11.36** the prosthesis has now been removed and the patient is left with a painless pseudoarthrosis; however, her gait is severely limited in view of the instability and shortening on that side.

11.37

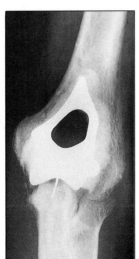

11.38

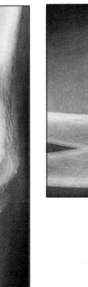

11.37, 11.38 This patient has an excellent result from a Souter–Strathclyde total elbow replacement. This is an unconstrained prosthesis with a metal humeral component cemented in place and this articulates with a polyethylene olecranon component cemented into the ulna. This prosthesis is suitable for rheumatoid arthritis and OA.

Joint allografts

Joint transplantation is not new. Eric Lexer reported on his results in 1908. Since then the use of allografts has been well-established in orthopaedic surgery. In the management of bone tumours satisfactory results in 84% at one year are reported (Manymneh *et al.*, 1985). However, results from Toronto in the treatment of OA have not been so encouraging, with only 42% being successful at six years (McDermott *et al.*, 1985). The results of transplantation to replace part of a joint after trauma have been better. Transplantation of total elbow allografts, used as a salvage procedure following trauma, have produced satisfactory results in seven out of 10 patients, aged between 20 and 64 years. The potential complication rate is high and the long-term results unknown (Urbaniak and Black, 1985). With the development of sophisticated tissue banks, the use of allografts in the treatment of OA may increase, but at present must be considered to be in its infancy (Imamalier, 1969).

Consideration of individual joints in the surgical management of OA

The spine

Osteoarthritis is extremely common both in the cervical and in the lower lumbar spine. Whilst movement of the spine is important, it is stability that is of utmost importance in order to protect the underlying spinal cord, as well as to supply resistance to gravitational forces. Therefore arthrodesis is the surgical treatment of choice. If successful, this provides excellent relief of pain, provided that the source of pain has been accurately identified – and this is extremely difficult. However, when one vertebral segment is totally immobilised, those above and below undergo excess stress and may develop degenerative change earlier than would otherwise have been expected. The surgical management then becomes more difficult in terms of how many segments should be fused (*see* **11.28**).

Replacement of the intervertebral disc with a plastic prosthesis can now be performed and the long-term results are awaited.

Sternoclavicular joint

Whilst OA is not uncommon in this joint, surgical intervention is unusual, but if required excision arthroplasty of the medial end of the clavicle produces pain relief, maintains movement and does not create any significant instability.

Acromioclavicular joint

Osteoarthritis is quite common radiologically, and when symptomatic produces pain through the abduction range of 130° to 180°. Inferior osteophyte formation may interfere with the function of the supraspinatus tendon. If an acromioplasty is being done for an impingement syndrome then it may also be necessary either to remove the osteophytes or excise the distal end of the clavicle. Excision arthroplasty is the treatment of choice for this joint.

Shoulder

Osteoarthritis of this joint is now known to occur much more frequently than previously realised. Arthrodesis has in the past been the surgical treatment of choice. This achieves pain relief, and motion around the shoulder girdle is maintained by the scapulothoracic articulation. In the young patient and those with paralysis of the shoulder, arthrodesis is still the treatment of choice. Neer (1974) advocated the use of a hemi-arthroplasty, which consisted of a hemisphere with a stem down the humeral shaft articulating with the glenoid cavity. Good pain relief was achieved in about 50% of patients, but the range of motion was extremely limited. Total arthroplasty of the shoulder joint is still in the developmental stage, but results are encouraging and it is an acceptable treatment for OA, and more particularly rheumatoid arthritis.

Elbow joint

Both stability and motion are required at the elbow joint. Excision arthroplasty has the advantage of maintaining motion, but there is loss of stability (Knight and Van Zandt, 1952). This prevents the patient from doing any heavy work but it can produce freedom from pain whilst maintaining the ability of the hand to reach the mouth. It would be essential for the opposite elbow to have some degree of stability in order to do heavier work. If the patient is required to use walking aids, then excisional arthroplasty has distinct disadvantages. However, Fisher reported 39 successful operations out of 45 elbows and the failures would appear to result from residual stiffness and pain (Fisher, 1973; Froimson et al. 1976) obtained good results in five patients by a fascial interpositional arthroplasty. Hemi-arthroplasties have been described but have not been successful. Arthrodesis, whilst being difficult to achieve, produces excellent stability and pain relief but its fixed position is a significant functional problem. Total elbow joint replacement has developed rapidly over the past decade and is now an accepted surgical procedure, mainly for rheumatoid arthritis. Souter has achieved excellent results using a prosthesis, the metal component of which simulates the shape of the lower end of the humerus and articulates with a polyethylene olecranon, which again is a similar shape to the proximal ulna (11.36, 11.37). This prosthesis has been used in patients with OA with considerable success. However the high stresses imposed by such patients may lead to a high failure rate in the long term.

In the patient with early OA of the elbow, debridement of the posterior osteophytes and loose bodies from the anterior compartment has been shown to be quite successful (Stanley and Winson, 1989). This can be achieved with minimal morbidity via a posterior approach. A foramen is cut in the olecranon fossa to gain access to the anterior compartment. The early results are very good.

The proximal radio-ulnar joint

Arthropathy of the proximal radio-ulnar joint is usually seen in rheumatoid arthritis. Osteoarthritis may develop as a result of trauma, particularly after fractures of the radial head with subsequent joint incongruity. The main complaint is loss of forearm rotation and if this is painful then surgical correction may be necessary. The most common form of surgical management is an excision arthroplasty. The radial head is excised leaving the orbicular ligament in place. Such an operation combined with synovectomy is extremely successful in the rheumatoid elbow. However, in the osteoarthritic joint in a relatively young, physically active person, then the results are not so satisfactory. There is some weakness of grip and rotation. There may also be shortening of the radius with subsequent painful disruption of the distal radio-ulnar joint, which may then require surgical treatment. An interposition arthroplasty using a silastic radial head may theoretically prevent the shortening of the radius, but the high compressive forces associated with a shearing stress across the surface of the silastic, may create silastic debris and subsequent small particle synovitis (11.39). There is no completely satisfactory surgical answer to the osteoarthritic proximal radio-ulnar joint.

Distal radio-ulnar joint

Arthritis at this joint is usually the result of rheumatoid disease and therefore excision of the distal end of the ulna and a synovectomy is extremely effective, i.e. excision arthroplasty. Osteoarthritis is usually associated with a fracture of the distal radius and may cause painful restriction of movement such as is seen in a malunited Colles' fracture. Once again excisional arthroplasty of the distal end of the ulna is quite a satisfactory operation in the elderly person who is not putting great demands on the wrist. In the younger manual worker some weakness of grip may result although, because of the absence of pain, the function of the hand may be better. The interposition of a piece of silastic over the end of the ulna does not appear to confer any benefit in this operation. In the younger patient, creation of a pseudoarthrosis just proximal to the distal end of the ulna may confer more stability to the wrist joint. This is described as a Suave-Kapandji operation (previously incorrectly known as a Laurenstein procedure). The distal end of the ulna is reduced into its correct position and arthrodesed to the distal end of the radius. Just proximal to this arthodesis a 1 cm segment of the ulna is excised, deliberately leading to the creation of a pseudoarthrosis which maintains rotation of the forearm. The distal end of the ulna, now arthrodesed to the radius, maintains stability on the ulnar side of the wrist joint (Sauve-Kapandji, 1936).

Radiocarpal joint

Primary OA of the wrist joint is uncommon and most degenerative wrists are secondary to trauma. The wrist may be painful and stiff, and the grip strength diminished producing significant disability in the physically active person. The restriction in function is not confined to manual workers, as even the firm grip required in shaking hands can produce sharp pain. Fractures of the distal radius involving the articular surface, malunion of the Colles' fracture, with malalignment of the carpal bones, ununited fractures of the scaphoid, Keinbock's disease of the lunate and various carpal instabilities caused by ligamentous damage may all lead to degenerative change (see **11.8**, **11.9**).

Total arthroplasty of the wrist joint has been successful in the rheumatoid patient (**11.40**). However, in the patient with an isolated radiocarpal problem and full elbow and hand function, the longevity of these prostheses is limited. The alternatives that exist include pseudoarthrosis, i.e. proximal row carpectomy, or arthrodesis. If it is essential to maintain some degree of wrist movement then proximal row carpectomy provides the solution, but there is some sacrifice in terms of grip strength. Function is surprisingly good with the patient taking approximately six months to achieve a final end result (Stamm, 1944).

If strength is essential, and flexion-extension of the wrist can be sacrificed, then arthrodesis is the treatment of choice. It is fixed either with a piece of cortical bone screwed across the dorsal surface or by plate fixation together with bone graft. Arthrodesis gives an excellent result, rotation is maintained and grip strength is powerful (**11.41**, **11.42**).

11.39

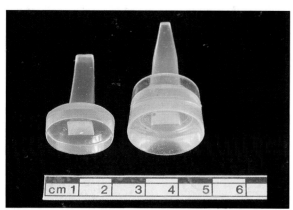

11.39 On the right is a silastic radial head replacement. Various sizes are available. The stem fits down the shaft of the radius. On the left is a silastic interposition arthroplasty for the great toe. This can also be used in the carpometacarpal joint of the thumb.

11

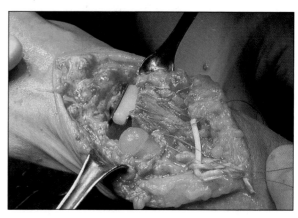

11.40 A Swanson silastic wrist joint lies between the distal end of the radius and the carpal bones. Titanium grommets separate the edge of the prosthesis from the underlying bone. A silastic replacement for the ulnar head is also seen in the lower half of the picture. This type of prosthesis is most suitable for rheumatoid arthritis.

11.41

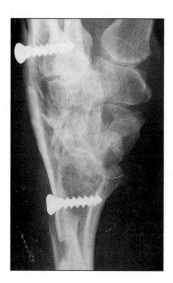
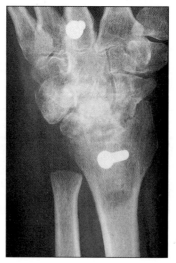

11.42

11.41, 11.42 An arthrodesis of the wrist is the treatment of choice for post-traumatic OA. This wrist has been fused by denuding the articular surface of the radius and the carpus of its articular cartilage and then stabilising this by screw fixation of a corticocancellous graft taken from the wing of the ilium. This will require plaster immobilisation but will give a sound arthrodesis allowing supination and pronation of the forearm. Mobility has been lost but stability is excellent and therefore the power grip of the hand is excellent.

The wrist is perhaps the one joint where neurectomy may be of value. The terminal branch of the posterior interosseous nerve is divided as it crosses the wrist joint. Further complete denervations have been described and there seems to be no problem in producing a Charcot-type joint. The long-term results of neurectomy are awaited.

Carpometacarpal (trapeziometacarpal) joint of the thumb

This is an extremely common joint in which to find radiographic and clinical osteoarthrosis (**11.43**, **11.44**). Conservative treatment is often quite successful. However, persistent pain and weakness of pinch grip are indications for surgical treatment. It is important, before considering surgery, to assess the state of the scaphotrapezial joint which also may be involved in the degenerative process. Excision and interposition arthroplasty are the two most common surgical procedures. With an excision arthroplasty the entire trapezium is removed and the space that is left fills with blood which is eventually replaced with fibrous tissue. The thumb is immobilised, maintaining length whilst this occurs. Pain relief is usually excellent but there is some weakness of pinch grip (Mulder, 1948).

Interposition arthroplasty may be performed using a rolled-up tendon. The flexor carpi radialis tendon is split longitudinally and one half is divided proximally but left attached to its insertion. It is then rolled up and placed within the vacant space (Fromison, 1970). A

silastic implant may be inserted to take the place of the trapezium with very good results (Swanson, 1985). Dislocation of the silastic prosthesis and occasional small particle synovitis are problems associated with this type of interposition arthroplasty (Gervis, 1973).

A total joint arthroplasty, similar to the hip joint prosthesis (i.e. a ball and socket) is available and has been quite successful in both rheumatoid and OA. Dislocation and loosening of the trapezial component can cause problems. The results of this de la Caffinière prosthesis do look promising (**11.45**).

Arthrodesis provides a very stable joint with excellent pain relief and maintenance of a good pinch grip (Stark *et al.*, 1977). Movement is limited, however, and it is difficult to place the hand flat on the table. It is important that the scaphotrapezial joint is not involved in any degenerative change. The operation is reserved for the younger patient whose physical demands are quite high (Carroll and Hill, 1973; Stark *et al.*, 1977).

11.43

11.44

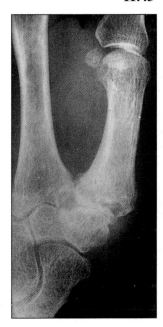
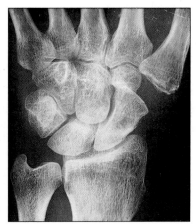

11.43, 11.44 Severe OA of the carpometacarpal joint of the thumb (**11.43**). This is an extremely common area in which to find OA which produces significant pain on all movements of the thumb and restricts pinch grip.

11.44 A trapeziectomy has been performed allowing pseudoarthrosis between the scaphoid and the first metacarpal. There is excellent painless movement but because of slight instability the pinch grip is weaker than normal, although better than that when the joint was painful.

11.45

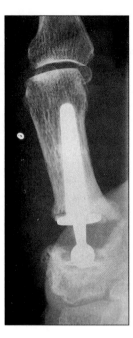

11.45 This is a de la Caffinière prosthesis used as a total joint replacement for the carpometacarpal joint of the thumb. The metal ball articulates with a polyethylene socket which is cemented into the trapezium.

Interphalangeal joints of the hand

The distal interphalangeal joint is a common site of degenerative change but is generally asymptomatic. If it becomes unstable then fusion is the treatment of choice. The proximal interphalangeal joint may become involved in isolated degenerative change, and if so then fusion achieves stability and strength on the radial side of the hand. However, on the ulnar side of the hand, flexion for grip may be more important, and therefore a flexible silastic prosthesis will maintain some movement.

The hip joint

The treatment of OA of the hip joint occupies a significant proportion of the operating time of the orthopaedic surgeon. It is the joint which has become successfully salvaged by surgery and rated as one of the top operations for improving the quality of patients' lives. Whilst total hip replacement is by far the most common method of surgical treatment, other forms of surgery have enjoyed popularity in the past and occasionally there is still a place for some of these procedures.

Denervation has been used with some success, but Hamblen (1975) found the results unpredictable and effective in terms of pain relief in less than 50% of cases. In very elderly and medically unfit patients, pain clinics may help by providing injection of the femoral, obturator and sciatic nerves with local anaesthetics. Drilling of the femoral neck, cheilectomy and muscle release operations are now seldom practised. Surgical procedures which still have

something to offer include osteotomy, arthrodesis and arthroplasty. Creation of a pseudoarthrosis should now be regarded as a salvage procedure for failed total hip replacements (*see* **11.33–11.36**).

Before the success of total hip arthroplasty the osteotomy was by far the most popular method of treatment. The reasons why it worked remain unclear, although the alteration of mechanical stress, change in the weight-bearing portion of the femoral head and an alteration to the blood supply are all factors which probably contributed. Nissen (1963) postulated that the osteotomy cut off the excessive blood supply, reducing the pain and this consequently caused a metabolic change and the joint remoulded. The osteotomy is performed in the intertrochanteric region and rigid internal fixation allows early mobility. The change in position that is achieved by the osteotomy is controversial. The European school has considered that accurate planning, based on radiographs, is absolutely essential, whereas the British school considered that the osteotomy was the most important part, together with some form of displacement which altered the mechanical axis and corrected the deformity. That the leg faced the front and came down straight was the most important aspect (Helfet, 1969). The development of a joint space was often seen after displacement osteotomies (**11.46**, **11.47**). Although the results were rather unreliable, it did provide excellent relief of pain for a considerable period of time for many patients.

Arthrodesis of the hip gives an excellent pain-free stable result and although not commonly practised today, still has a place in the treatment of the young, vigorous adult, with post-traumatic degenerative disease of the hip. A prolonged period of immobilisation has been required in the past, but methods of rigid internal fixation have allowed early mobility (**11.48**). It is possible to convert an arthrodesed hip to a total joint arthroplasty in later years if adjacent joints become degenerate.

By far the most popular surgical procedure for OA of the hip is total joint replacement. This involves the replacement of the acetabulum by a plastic cup, with or without metal backing, fixed to the pelvis either by bone cement or by allowing bone to grow into the prosthesis in the cementless variety. A ball with a stem, representing the head of the femur, is inserted into the shaft of the femur and again either held there by bone cement or by allowing bone in-growth to occur into the prosthesis. Considerable controversy still exists as to the best method of fixing the prosthesis to the bone, but either way excellent results can be achieved, producing a 95% chance of a successful outcome (Dobbs, 1980). The indication for surgery is pain, especially pain at rest. Stiffness of the hip without pain is not a good indication for surgery unless both hip joints are involved and the position of the stiffened joint causes difficulty with function. In ankylosing spondylitis, the bilateral involvement of hip joints producing inability to abduct may, in the absence of pain, be a good indication for surgery. Advanced age should not be considered a barrier for surgical intervention as an elderly patient's life may be totally transformed by the relief of pain from the hip, giving them the ability to walk around and remain independent. Caution has to be exercised in the younger patient whose demands are obviously greater than those in their eighth decade of life and in whom a

11.46

11.47

11.48

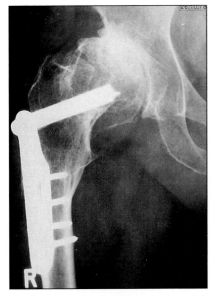
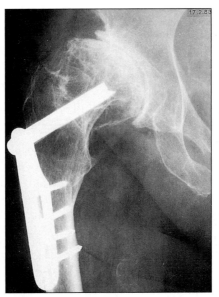
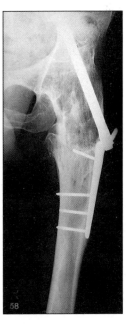

11.46, 11.47 An intertrochanteric osteotomy has been performed for OA of the hip (**11.46**). Five years later (**11.47**) the patient is asymptomatic and the joint space has been restored. It is not the change in position of the femoral head that has given the appearance of this restoration of joint space but either a change in mechanical forces or a change in the blood supply has allowed regeneration of a cartilage space. Both joint mobility and stability have been maintained.

11.48 Arthrodesis of the hip has been performed using a method of internal fixation. The joint will be totally pain-free, stable but immobile.

greater longevity of prosthesis is required, yet in whom the prosthesis will be put under greater stress during its lifetime. As a result of various complications, it is possible to leave the patient worse off than they were with their osteoarthritic hip. All patients have to be warned that revision surgery may be necessary and the success rate from the revision is lower and the complication rate twice that of the primary intervention. Approximately 40 000 hip replacements are performed in the UK each year and as the numbers increase and each year goes by, the number requiring revision surgery will increase. Some practices claim that over half of all the hip replacements are revisions, which are more complicated, more time-consuming and more expensive.

Infection has been of great concern since the original hip replacements were inserted earlier this century. The introduction of the clear-air operating theatre, the administration of antibiotics during the operation and the inclusion of antibiotics within the bone cement are factors which have helped to reduce the infection rate to as low as 0.5%. Infection rates do, however, vary and have been reported as high as 11%.

Thromboembolism is a significant cause of mortality and morbidity, with a reported incidence of between 30% and 70%, and the incidence of fatal pulmonary embolism varying between 1% and 4%. Physical and pharmacological methods of prevention have been well tried but so far no single method has been shown conclusively to prevent fatal pulmonary emboli following hip replacement, although some methods purport to show a decrease in the incidence of venous thrombosis.

Dislocation of the hip joint can be a problem, especially in the uncooperative patient or one with neuromuscular problems. Fracture of the femur may occur peroperatively or after a simple fall at any time postoperatively, usually at the lower end of the prosthesis. These can usually be treated by internal fixation (**11.49**, **11.50**).

Loosening of the prosthesis is a major long-term problem which usually necessitates revision. It may be the result of a low-grade deep infection which can be difficult to differentiate from aseptic loosening, the reasons for which remain controversial (**11.51**). Excessive thinning of the proximal femoral cortex occurs resulting in fracture either before or during surgical reconstruction. A salvage solution includes the insertion of a large prosthesis which gains a grip in the distal femur and copious bone-graft is packed around the proximal femur.

Ectopic bone may occur around the upper femur, producing marked stiffness. Neurovascular complications may occur during surgery and, in particular, the sciatic nerve is vulnerable.

Fracture of the stem of the prosthesis has been a problem in the past but the advancement in metallurgy has virtually eliminated this complication (*see* **11.51**).

11.49

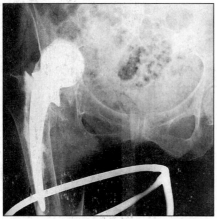

11.50

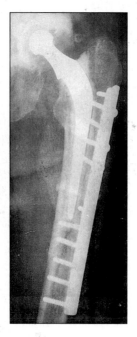

11.

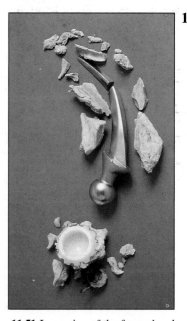

11.49, 11.50 A hemiarthroplasty (**11.49**) has been performed. The hard metal ball has burrowed its way through the acetabulum and now protrudes into the pelvis. This will have to be removed and a total hip replacement performed. A successful Charnley total hip replacement (**11.50**) has been complicated by a fracture of the shaft of the femur at the tip of the prosthesis. There is a significant change in stiffness of the bone at this level where the femur is susceptible to fracture. The fracture has been internally fixed using a plate and the prosthesis remains in place. The outcome was successful.

11.51 Loosening of the femoral and acetabular components can occur even when they are cemented in place with acrylic cement. It has been necessary here to remove both components. The femoral stem has broken and the cement has fractured into several fragments. Loosening of the prosthesis produces pain.

Knee joint

Surgical treatment of OA of the knee offers several options. Debridement has been popular and the operation used by Pridie involved a wide arthrotomy, removal of excess osteophytes, loose cartilage fragments and degenerate menisci, then the subchondral bone was drilled in areas where it was exposed. The operation appeared to halt the progress of the disease and was fairly successful in terms of pain relief (Insall *et al.*, 1974;) (*see* **11.19–11.21**).

Despite that success, the operation is now rarely performed, although debridement and lavage by arthroscopic techniques are popular at present. The results seem to be short-lived and this could be regarded as a holding procedure in the younger patient, alleviating symptoms until the patient is older and requires a more definitive procedure. Lavage is useful for crystal arthropathy.

Localised areas of loss of articular cartilage around the subchondral bone can be quite successfully treated by the implantation of a plug of woven carbon-fibre. This appears to act as scaffolding for the development of fibrocartilage and the short-term results seem impressive (Muckle, 1990) (**11.52–11.54**). Arthrodesis

of the knee is now seldom used in the treatment of OA, although it remains an option for the treatment of difficult cases and failed total knee arthroplasty. It produces a painless stable knee but nowadays patients find the subsequent disability and cosmetic result unacceptable when they compare themselves with those patients who have had total knee replacements (Frymoyer and Hoaglund, 1974).

Before the success of the total knee arthroplasty, the osteotomy was the mainstay of surgical treatment. It is particularly successful when there is a varus or even a valgus deformity. There are limitations to the degree of deformity that can be corrected, and it is suggested that there should be no more than 20° of fixed flexion with ability to flex at least 90°, and that there should be no more than 15° of varus deformity (Insall, 1974; Jackson *et al.*, 1969). Coventry (1973) performed an upper tibial as well as a lower femoral osteotomy and obtained very good results. The degree of deformity can be easily measured by taking anteroposterior radiographs of the entire leg in the weight-bearing position. Osteotomies are created which bring the centre of the hip joint, the centre of

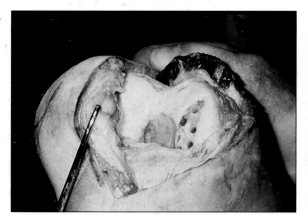

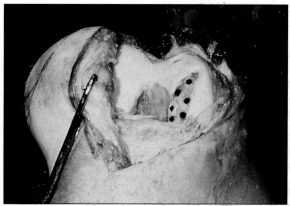

11.52, 11.53 An area of the femoral condyle has been denuded of its degenerative articular cartilage. Multiple small drill holes have been made similar to those in the 'Pridie' procedure. In **11.53** the holes have now been filled with rods of carbon fibre ('Medicarb' manufactured by Surgicraft Ltd., England. Acknowledgement Mr J. Betts, Gateshead.)

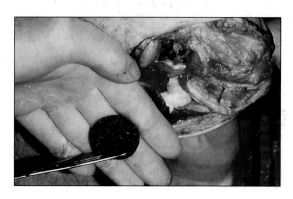

11.54 When large areas of articular cartilage have been lost a pad of carbon fibre can be inserted.

the knee and the centre of the ankle all within the same vertical line (**11.55**, **11.56**). For the young patient with medial compartment OA associated with the varus deformity, upper tibial osteotomy is probably still the treatment of choice. In the older patient with a similar problem, a unicondylar knee replacement may be more satisfactory (Broughton *et al.*, 1986; Thornhill and Scott, 1989). In this situation the surface of one femoral condyle is replaced by a metal component and the tibial plateau is replaced by a polythylene component.

When both the medial and the lateral compartments of the knee joint are involved in degenerative change, then by far the most popular surgical treatment is a total knee replacement. There is a choice in the principle of the prosthesis. It may be a totally constrained prosthesis, i.e. the two components are joined by a hinge (**11.57**). It may be semiconstrained, in which case there is no direct linkage between the two prostheses but the design entails a degree of interlocking. The unconstrained prosthesis replaces the condyles of the femur and the tibia with prostheses of similar shape to the normal anatomy. Usually a metal prosthesis covers the lower end of the femur and the tibial component is made of a high-density polyethylene. There are many designs of these condylar prostheses, some allowing the cruciate ligaments to be retained and others sacrificing them. The 'Oxford' knee has two mobile 'menisci' inserted between the femoral and tibial components. Refinement of the total knee replacement is still taking place; however, the condylar knee replacements are doing extremely well and success rates are starting to match those of total hip replacement (**11.58–11.61**).

The usual problems of prosthetic insertion can be encountered, but of particular concern around the knee joint is the poor wound healing and consequent infection which can become a significant problem. An above-knee amputation is not unknown when one of these infections gets out of hand.

Following femorotibial replacement, patellofemoral pain and lateral subluxation of the patella can be a problem. Controversy exists as to whether an implant should be placed on the under-surface of the patella to allow it to glide freely over the femoral condyles (**11.62**, **11.63**).

11.55   **11.56**   **11.57**

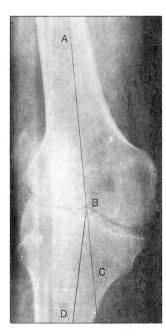
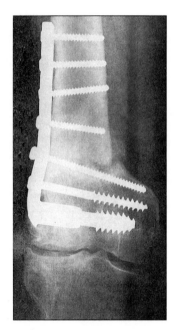
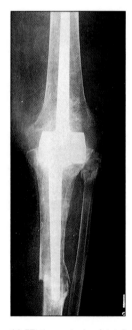

11.55, 11.56 Osteoarthritis of the lateral femorotibial compartment is present secondary to trauma (**11.55**). The line A–B–C joins the centre of the femoral head to the centre (B) of the knee join. This line A–C will pass medial to the ankle joint. Line B–D joins the centre of the knee to the centre of the ankle joint. The angle D–B–C indicates the degree of valgus. When planing the supracondylar osteotomy, the aim will be to bring the line B–D to overlie B–C. In **11.56** the supracondylar osteotomy has been performed and internally fixed. The joint space is now apparent on the lateral side and the patient is significantly improved. The stress on this joint is now evenly distributed between the medial and lateral joint compartments.

11.57 A constrained total knee replacement showing one of the complications, i.e. a fracture of the tibia at the tip of the prosthesis.

11.58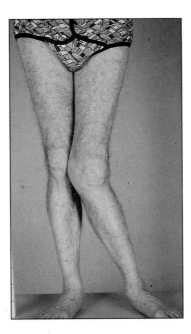

11.59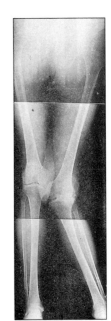

11.60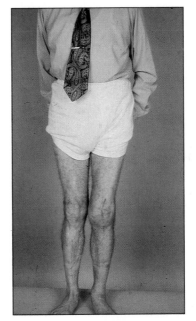

11.61

11.58–11.61 The patient has a severe valgus deformity associated with OA of the lateral compartment of the knee joint (**11.58**). Weight-bearing films show the gross malalignment of the knee (**11.59**). A line joining the centre of the femoral head to the centre of the knee joint would pass medial to the ankle joint. Following a total knee replacement, the alignment is satisfactory and the patient is happy (**11.60**). The radiograph now shows a better alignment of the knee joint (**11.61**) and a line passing from the femoral head to the centre of the knee joint passes through the centre of the ankle. (Acknowledgement Mr J. H. Newman, Bristol.)

11.62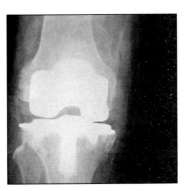

11.63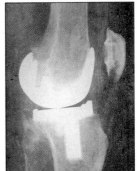

11.62, 11.63 An unconstrained total knee replacement with a polyethylene component cemented to the upper surface of the patella.

Patellofemoral joint

The patellofemoral joint may be involved with OA in isolation. This can occur as a result of trauma. Probably the most common operation has been the creation of pseudoarthrosis, i.e. a patellectomy. Results of this procedure have been acceptable, with 80% having good results, although the cosmetic aspect may not be attractive to female patients (Ackroyd, 1978; French, 1959).

Osteotomy of the patella has been used to alleviate pain (Macnicol, 1985). An elaboration of the osteotomy is to reduce the force transmitted across the kneecap by compression against the underlying femoral condyle. To this end Maquet (1976) has designed an osteotomy in which the tibial tuberosity is elevated by approximately 2 cm. This alters the mechanical lever-arm above the knee joint and reduces the compression force on the patella as the knee goes into flexion. Maquet only performs this operation when there is underlying subchondral sclerosis demonstrated in the patella. However, this particular operation has been used for treatment of patellofemoral pain without radiological change and the results are not as impressive. The problem with the operation is the resulting prominence of the tibial tuberosity, which makes kneeling difficult and can be cosmetically unacceptable.

A hemiprosthesis, i.e. replacement of the underlying surface of the kneecap, is the other surgical possibility. This form of surgery is still perhaps in its infancy and has not been widely accepted.

Ankle joint

In principle there are two operations which are helpful for OA of the ankle joint. Arthrodesis has enjoyed a huge success with minimal resultant disability and excellent relief of pain. The position of arthrodesis is important. In the male it is best placed in the plantigrade position and in the female there should be a few degrees of equinus, depending on the footwear that is normally worn. Compensatory movements occur at the midtarsal joint and patients who have had this operation often demonstrate a relatively normal gait.

Total arthroplasty of the ankle has been quite sucessful in the patient with rheumatoid arthritis, but its long-term role in the treatment of OA has yet to be evaluated. Once again it is the high stress placed through the joint in the younger patient with single joint involvement which causes the concern associated with loosening of this prosthesis.

Midtarsal joint

Osteoarthritis may occur in the midtarsal joints of the foot as well as in the subtalar joints. These are all best treated by arthrodesis.

First metatarsophalangeal joint

This is an extremely common joint for OA. In the younger patient it presents as pain associated with restriction of dorsiflexion. This is often seen in footballers. Here cheilectomy may be of great value. The dorsal osteophytes are removed together with a dorsal wedge of bone and this reduces the impingement of the proximal phalanx during the push-off phase of gait. Mobility as well as stability are maintained and pain is significantly reduced. The patient must be warned that recurrence of osteophytes can occur.

In younger patients the other popular procedure is arthrodesis. This produces stability and relief of pain. However, it is preferable to have some dorsiflexion movement of the interphalangeal joint of the great toe in order to allow push-off to occur. The position of arthrodesis is crucial, as too much plantar flexion will cause excess weight-bearing under the interphalangeal joint, and excessive dorsiflexion may produce pain under the metatarsal head.

In older patients and those not putting a great demand on the foot, then interposition arthroplasty can be quite successful. Silastic is the popular material at present. An excisional arthroplasty, i.e. Keller's operation, is also helpful, but it does tend to defunction the great toe, which in the younger patient may be a disability, especially if they have any athletic desires.

Summary

The aim of surgical treatment of OA is to relieve pain, maintain or restore motion and maintain or restore stability. A number of surgical procedures are available and each joint and each patient has to be considered individually. The surgeon must make a recommendation taking into consideration many factors. A man-made artificial joint must never be considered the equivalent of a normal joint, either in its function or its longevity. It is important that the patient is also made aware of these limitations. By far the best treatment of OA is its prevention.

References and further reading

Ackroyd, C.E., Polyzoides, A.J. (1978) Patellectomy for osteoarthritis. *J. Bone Joint Surg.*, **60B**, 353–357.

Agerholn–Christensen, J., Gleave, J.R.W. (1956) Drilling of the osteoarthritic hip. *Proc. R. Soc. Med.*, **49**, 964–965.

Anoldi, C., Lemperg, R.K., Linderholm, H. (1975) Intraosseous hypertension and pain in the knee. *J. Bone Joint Surg.*, **57B**, 360–363.

Bateman, J.E. (1948) Denervation of the elbow joint for relief of pain. *J. Bone Joint Surg.*, **30B**, 635.

Burwell, H.W., Charnley, A.D. (1965) The treatment of displaced fractures of the ankle by rigid internal fixation and early joint movement. *J. Bone Joint Surg.*, **47B**, 637–660.

Broughton, N.S., Newman, J.H., Baily, R.A.J. (1986) Unicompartmental replacement and high tibial osteotomy for osteoarthritis of the knee. *J. Bone Joint Surg.*, **64B**, 447–452.

Bucholz, H.W., Elson, R.A., Engelbrecht, E., Lodenkämper, H., Röttger, J., Siegel, A. (1981) Management of deep infection of total hip replacement. *J. Bone Joint Surg.*, **63B**, 342–353.

Carroll, R.E., Hill, N.A. (1973) Arthrodesis of the carpometacarpal joint of the thumb. *J. Bone Joint Surg.*, **55B**, 292–294.

Carter, P.R., Benton, L.J., Dysert, P.A. (1986) Silicone rubber carpal implants, a study of the incidence of late osseous complications. *J. Hand Surg.*, **11A**, 639–644.

Casagrande, P.A., Austin, B.P., Indek, W. (1951) Denervation of the ankle joint. *J. Bone Joint Surg.*, **33A**, 723–730.

Charnley, J. (1961) Arthroplasty of the hip. A new operation. *Lancet*, **i**, 1129–1132.

Citron, N., Neil, M. (1987) Dorsal wedge of the proximal phalanx for hallux rigidus. *J. Bone Joint Surg.*, **69B**, 835–857.

Coventry, M.B. (1973) Osteotomy about the knee for degenerative and rheumatoid arthritis. *J. Bone Joint Surg.*, **55A**, 23–48.

Crabbe, W.A. (1964) Excision of the proximal row of the carpus. *J. Bone Joint Surg.*, **46B**, 708–711.

Dobbs, H.S. (1980) Survivorship of total hip replacements. *J. Bone Joint Surg.*, **62B**, 168–173.

Epstein, H.C. (1974) Posterior fracture-dislocation of the hip. *J. Bone Joint Surg.*, **56A**, 1103–1127.

Fisher, D.B. (1973) Excisional elbow arthroplasty. *J. Bone Joint Surg.*, **55A**, 1305.

French, P.R. (1959) The patellofemoral joint. *J. Bone Joint Surg.*, **41B**, 857.

Froimson, A.I., Silva, J.E., Richey, de E.G. (1976) Cutis arthropathy of the elbow joint. *J. Bone Joint Surg.*, **58A**, 863–865.

Fromison, A.I. (1970) Tendon arthroplasty of the trapeziometacarpal joint. *Clin. Orthopaed. Rel. Res.*, **70**, 191–199.

Frymoyer, J.W., Hoaglund, F.T. (1974) The role of arthrodesis in reconstruction of the knee. *Clin. Orthopaed. Related Res.*, **101**, 82–92.

Gervis, W.H. (1949) Excision of the trapezium for osteoarthritis of the trapeziometacarpal joint. *J. Bone Joint Surg.*, **31B**, 537–539.

Gervis, W.H. (1973) A review of excision of the trapezium for osteoarthritis of the trapeziometacarpal joint after 25 years. *J. Bone Joint Surg.*, **55B**, 56–57.

Girdlestone, G.R., Watson-Jones, R., MacFarland, B., Stamm, T.T. Priddie, K.H. (1945) *Proc. R. Soc. Med.*, **38**, 363.

Haggart, G.E. (1940) The surgical treatment of degenerative arthritis of the knee joint. *J. Bone Joint Surg.*, **22**, 717–729.

Hamblen, D.L. (1975) In *Surgical Management of Degenerative Arthritis of the Lower Limb*. Cruess R.L., Mitchell, N.S. (Eds). 65–78. Philadelphia, Lea and Febiger.

Helal, B. (1965) The pain in primary osteoarthritis of the knee. *Postgrad. Med. J.*, **41**, 172–181.

Helfet, A.J. (1969) Concept of arrest of osteoarthritis in the hip and knee. In *Recent Advances in Orthopaedics*. Apley A.G. (Ed.). J & A Churchill Ltd, London, 361–375.

Imamaliev, A.S. (1969) Transplantation of articular bone ends. In *Recent Advances in Orthopaedics*. Apley, A.G. (Ed.). J & A Churchill Ltd, London., 209–263

Inglis, A.E., Jones, E.L. (1977) Proximal row carpectomy for disease of the proximal row. *J. Bone Joint Surg.*, **59A**, 460–463.

Insall, J., Shoji, H., Mayer, V. (1974) High tibial osteotomy. *J. Bone Joint Surg.*, **56A**, 1397–1405.

Insall, J.N. (1967) Intra-articular surgery for degenerative arthritis of the knee. A report of the work of the late K.H. Pridie. *J. Bone Joint Surg.*, **49B**, 211–228.

Jackson, J.P., Waugh, W., Green, J.P. (1969) High tibial osteotomy for osteoarthritis of the knee. *J. Bone Joint Surg.*, **51B**, 88–94.

Johnson, L.L. (1986) Arthroscopic abrasion arthroplasty. *Arthroscopy*, **2** (1), 54.

Kaplan, E.D. (1948) Resection of obturator nerve for relief of pain in arthritis of the hip joint. *J. Bone Joint Surg.*, **30A**, 213.

Kestler, O.C. (1946) A surgical procedure for the painful arthritic hand. *Bull. Hosp. Joint Dis.*, **7**, 114.

Knight, R.A., Van Zandt, I.L. (1952) Arthroplasty of the elbow. *J. Bone Joint Surg.*, **34A**, 610–612.

Law, W.A. (1948) Postoperative study of vitallium mold arthroplasty of the hip joint. *J. Bone Joint Surg.*, **30B**, 76.

Leach, R.E. (1963) Femoral cortical drilling for relief of pain due to degenerative arthritis of the hip. *J. Bone Joint Surg.*, **45A**, 509–512.

Lexer, E. (1908) Joint transplantation. *Clin. Orthopaed. Rel. Res.*, 197, 4–10 (1985). (Translation from UEDER, *Gelenktransplantation, Ned. Clin.*, 1908, **4**, 817.

Mackenzie, J.F. (1936) Osteoarthritis of the hip and knee. Description of a surgical treatment. *Br. Med. J.*, **1**, 306–308.

Macnicol, M.F. (1985) Patellar osteotomy for intractable anterior knee pain. *J. Bone Joint Surg.*, **67B**, 156.

Magnuson, P.B. (1946) Technique of debridement of the knee joint for arthritis. *Surg. Clin. N. Am.*, **26**, 249.

Manymneh, W. Malinin, T.I., Mailley, J.T., Dick, H.M. (1985) Massive osteoarticular allografts in the reconstruction of extremities following resection of tumours not requiring chemotherapy and radiation. *Clin. Orthopaed. Rel. Res.*, **197**, 76–87.

Maquet, P. (1976) Advancement of the tibial tuberosity. *Clin. Orthopaed. Rel. Res.*, **115**, 225–229.

McDermott, A.G.B., Langer, F., Pritzker, K.P.H., Gross, A.E. (1985) Fresh small-fragment osteochondral allografts. *Clin. Orthopaed. Rel. Res.*, **197**, 96–102.

McElwaine, J.P., Colville, J. (1984) Excision arthroplasty for infected total hip replacements. *J. Bone Joint Surg.*, **66B**, 168–171.

Muckle, D.S., Minns, R.J. (1990) Biological response to woven carbon fibre pads in the knee. *J. Bone Joint Surg.*, **72B**, 60–62.

Mulder, J.D. (1948) Denervation of the hip joint in osteoarthritis. *J. Bone Joint Surg.*, **30B**, 446.

Murley, A.H.G. (1960) Excision of the trapezium in osteoarthritis of the first carpometacarpal joint. *J. Bone Joint Surg.*, **42B**, 502–507.

Neer, C.S. Replacement arthroplasty for gleno-humeral osteoarthritis. *J. Bone & Joint Surgery*, **56A**, 1–13.

Neviaser, R.J. Proximal row carpectomy for post-traumatic disorders of the carpus. *J. Hand Surg.*, **8**, 301–305.

Nissen, K.I. The arrest of early primary osteoarthritis of the hip by osteotomy. *Proc. Roy. Soc. Med.*, **56**, 1051–1060.

O'Malley, A.G. Osteoarthritis of the hip. *J. Bone Joint Surg.*, **41B**, 888–889.

Obletz, B.E., Lockie, L.M., Milch E., and Hyman, I. Early effects of partial sensory denervation of the hip for relief of pain in chronic arthritis. *J. Bone Joint Surg.*, **31A**, 805–814.

Pridie, K.H. (1959) A method of resurfacing osteoarthritic knee joints. *J. Bone Joint Surg.*, **41B**, 618–619.

Rock, M.G. and Bourne, R.B. Excision arthroplasty of the hip. *J. Bone Joint Surg.*, **63B**, 457.

Rogan, M. A personal communication. Symposium on Arthroscopy. Harrogate 1989.

Salter, R.B., Simmonds, D.F., Malcolm, B.W., Rumble, E.J., MacMichael, D., Clements, M.D. (1980) The biological effects of continuous passive motion on the healing of full thickness defects in articular cartilage. *J. Bone Joint Surg.*, **62A**, 1232–1251.

Sauve-Kapandji. (1936) Nouvelle technique traitement chirurgical des luxations recidivantes isolées de l'extremitie inférieure du cubitus. *Journal de chirurgie*, **47**, 589–594.

Schonholtz, G.J. (1989) Arthroscopic debridement of the knee joint. *Orthopaed. Clin. N. Am.*, **20**, 257–263.

Smith-Petersen, M.N. (1939) Arthroplasty of the hip. A new method. *J. Bone Joint Surg.*, **21**, 269.

Solomon, L. (1981) Idiopathic necrosis of the femoral head. Pathogenesis and treatment. *Canadian J. Surg.*, **24**, 573–578.

Stamm, T.T. (1944) Excision of the proximal row of the carpus. *Proc. R. Soc. Med.*, **38**, 74.

Stanley, D., Winson, I.G. (1989) Osteoarthritis of the elbow. A more effective surgical approach. *J. Bone Joint Surg.*, **71B**, 874.

Stark, H.H., Moore, J.F., Ashworth, C.R., Boyes, J.H. (1977) Fusion of the first metacarpotrapezial joint for degenerative arthritis. *J. Bone Joint Surg.*, **59A**, 22–26.

Swanson, A.B., de Groot, G. (1985) Arthroplasty of the thumb base joints. *Clin. Orthopaed. Rel. Res.*, **195**, 151–160.

Thornhill, T.S., Scott, R.D. (1989) Unicompartmental total knee arthroplasty. *Orthopaed. Clin. N. Am.*, **20**, 245–255.

Urbaniak, J.R., Black, K.E. (1985) Cadaveric elbow allografts. *Clin. Orthopaed. Rel. Res.*, **197**, 131–140.

Wertheimer, L.G. (1952) The sensory nerves of the hip joint. *J. Bone Joint Surg.*, **34A**, 477–487.

Zizic, T.M., Hungerford, D.S. (1985) Osteonecrosis of bone. In *Textbook of Rheumatology*. 2nd ed. Kelly, W.N. (Ed.), W.B. Saunders, Philadelphia.

Index

loose bodies, 52
pain
    epidemiology, 18
    and radiographic evidence of OA, 18, 112
pattern of involvement, 11, 20
physiology
    materials, 40
    shape, 38–39
remodelling of, 38–39
shape
    and function, 29
    morbid anatomy, 41–42
    and physiology, 38–39
    as predisposing factor, 25, 26
stability exercises, 144
Joint space narrowing, 16, 17, 86–89

K

Kashin–Beck disease, 123–125
Keinbock's disease, 183
Keller's joint, 183
Kellgren and Lawrence grading system, 16–17, 86, 163
Keratan sulphate, 35, 44
Knee, 20
    arthrodesis, 180, 181, 192
    arthroplasty, 183
        osteotomy compared to, 151
    cartilage erosions, 43
    chondrocalcinosis, 76, 94, 154
    crystal deposition, 12, 74–76
    debridement, 178
    destructive OA, 98
    dysplasia, 100–101
    eburnation, 178
    effusion, 151
    lavage and abrasion arthroplasty, 179, 195
    ligament strains, 25, 57, 146, 152
    management
        periarticular problems, 152
        quadriceps exercises, 150–151
        trauma and development of OA, 150
        walking aids/splints, 151
    meniscal tears, 25, 107, 116, 150
    meniscectomy, 9, 25, 150
    morbidity and mortality, 62, 73
    natural history of OA, 73
    and obesity, 23, 147
    osteotomy, 151, 195–196
    pain
        and epidemiology, 18
        and radiographic change, 61
    patterns of OA, 73
    peri-articular problems, 152
    predisposing factors, 9, 73
    prevalence of OA, 21
    regression of OA, 113
    repetitive activity, 27
    scintiscanning, 105–106
    shape, 26, 30
    signs of OA, 62–63
    total arthroplasty, 186, 195, 196
    trauma to, and OA, 25, 57

windswept, 76

L

Laser therapy, 144
Leisure activities, 9, 27
Leucocyte count, 116
Ligament, 37, 152
    injury and OA, 57
    injury and repair, 52
    trauma-related lesion, management, 142
Light microscopy, polarised, 116
Lipopolysaccharide, 47
Loading
    and effect on physiology, 40
    elastic deformation due to, 30
    and joint shape, 38
    matrix structure and mechanical properties, 37
    obesity and OA, 23
    stress films, 87–88
Local anaesthetics, 192
Loose bodies, 52
Lumbar spine, 80, 180, 188

M

McKee–Farrar total hip replacement, 184–185
McMurray displacement osteotomy, 179
Magnetic resonance imaging (MRI), 37, 107–113, 163
Marble bone (Albers-Schonberg disease), 24
Marble bone appearance, 128
Marfan's syndrome, 142
Massage, 156
Matrilysin, 49
Matrix metalloproteinases, 48–50
Medical management, 141–156
    daily living, 143
    differential diagnosis of pain, 141
    exercises for muscle strength and joint stability, 144
    general patient approach, 141
    joint hyperlaxity, 142
    periarticular soft tissue lesions, 142
    psychological factors, 142
    radiographic appearance and symptoms, 141
    secondary OA, 143
    social factors, 142
Meniscal tears, 25, 107, 116, 150
Meniscectomy, 9, 25, 150
Menopause, 24
Meralgia paraesthetica, 153
Metabolic arthropathies, 129–133
Metacarpophalangeal joint
    CPPD deposition, 74, 76
    excisional arthroplasty, 183
    in haemochromatosis, 129
    second/third, 80, 81
Metalloproteinases, matrix, 48–50
Metatarsal rocker bar, 153
Metatarsophalangeal joint of big toe
    excisional arthroplasty, 183
    osteophyte, 41
Methyl-methacrylate cement, 185
Midtarsal joint, 198